Out Of My Head

My Journey Back from the Brain Tumor

Josie Blaine
12/22/2018

Acknowledgements

For centuries, people have taken their prayers to the Western Wall of Jerusalem. It is the last remaining wall of the Temple. Prayers for healing, marriage, children, or release from financial burden are written on slips of paper and wedged in the cracks of the wall. God hears them all.

These days, a quick Google or Twitter search will enable you to send your own prayer to be printed out at the wall. Technology has made our lives so easy.

Several years ago, my friend Diane was headed on a dream trip to the Holy Land. I was able to send my slip of prayer with her to the Western Wall, and I did so in every language I could think of. She retrieved my slip of paper on her way to the airport, one night as I was starting my radio show.

"Thank you. Merci. Efcharisto. Grazi. Gracias. Danke."

I believe that if God doesn't see our slips of paper, He hears the gratitude in our hearts.

My parents taught me to say thank you. They instilled

in me the love of things that last—friendships, cars, furniture, and people. It makes sense to invest in, do the work, and care for relationships. As I sit here, surrounded by hundreds of envelopes and pages of letters and notes from the fall of 1999, I can tell you, I feel I invest well.

I am thankful for every card, letter, every sunflower, bird of paradise, rose, stuffed animal, and every visit from dear friends to cheer me during days when I couldn't speak for myself.

Taylor Tehas, thank you for being so brave, and a good driver. Caroline Devine and Virgil Thompson, and everyone at Cox Radio/ San Antonio, thank you for being so wonderful. My adoration for our radio family is unspeakable. Ric, thank you for recognizing the critical dizziness I was trying to cover. To BK, for being the "work brother," always looking out for me, and Robert for keeping the music going.

Thank you, PA Larry Tatum and Dr. Ernesto Garza-Vale, along with Northeast Baptist Hospital, for the cheerful intake and the quickly getting me to the right place. Thank you for knowing where to find the care I would need.

I have a deep appreciation for the encouragers. My most heartfelt appreciation to the unparalleled Dr.

Christopher Bogaev, who went inside my head more than once, and came back out again. I am so thankful for the University of Texas Health Science Center of San Antonio, who participates in miracles every day. To Jennifer West and her staff of award-winning nurses: thank you for all you do on a daily basis for people who cannot help themselves.

My heart bursts with love and appreciation for Warm Springs Rehabilitation System, for helping me to quite literally walk, talk, feed and dress myself again. The memories I have of the faces I met in those hallways and gymnasiums will stay with me forever. My prayer is the work you do will inspire more people to help others.

Charolette, Nori, Adriana, Beto, Ken and Lorenzo, thank you forever.

I keep these cards and letters, and sometimes I reread beautiful words scrawled to encourage me, at a time when these words could have been each writer's goodbye. It is so special to witness this outpouring of love in my life.

"You saw your funeral," my mother told me. "Not many people get to see that."

Twenty-six letters are not enough to express to my

mother, who sat by my side and faced me with love every day I was motionless, thank you again and again. Thank you for feeding me, holding my hand, and for being there to help me stand again. Thank you, Daddy, for being so strong. To Maj. Gen. Floyd Baker (ret.) and Dolly, Johnny and Dee Wright, Jan Groen, The Coles Family, Chaplains Harris and Benson, Frank and Martha Connor, and the Fort Sam Houston Gift Chapel, thank you for being our family away from North Dakota.

Carrie, Tanya, Heather and Amanda, thank you for journeying all the way across the country to make sure I was okay.

Dear Southwest Methodist Hospital, and Texas Neurosciences Institute, I know I'm not the only one who believes miracles happen within your walls. Thank you to the nurses, the office staff, Dr. J. S. Luther of the Program PICANTE, and Neurosurgical Associates of San Antonio.

This book began immediately after I got out of the hospital, when someone said, "Write it down, so you don't forget." To that person: thank you. Mary Jane Rushlow suggested publishing it in 2001. Thank you. I take a little time sometimes.

To Pam Brinkworth Rutyna, whose mother is a brain tumor angel, I grieve your loss and thank you for your help. A portion of the proceeds of Out of My Head will be headed to the American Brain Tumor Association and St. Jude Children's Research Hospital.

I have a great family and am always surrounded by the most amazing souls. I don't take that for granted for a moment. Each of you is a unique blessing to me.

I believe we can't get through life alone, and God sends us whom we need. Thank you to my dear, dear friends who've become family. My family of coworkers through the years, have driven me and watched me closely through the seizures. some of you have listened to me perseverate on subjects beyond my control, most of you have continued to encourage me, despite pain, slowness, win, lose, or draw. Maybe you drank gallons of coffee with me and listened to my stories. You are in my heart.

Last but not least, my tech crew. Kirk, Doug, Trav, Megan, Nicole. if I beg you for technical mercy you're usually right there. Thank you.

CHAPTER ONE

I've told this story so many times, I feel like I'm quoting myself. I even laugh at the same places, and every listener looks at me, wide-eyed with horror or humor. Let me assure you, this is a story with a happy ending. I must write it down now, to get some of this out of my head.

Why do we tell our stories?

Well, I believe we are all human beings helping each other through life, toward Heaven. Wouldn't it be boring trying to bumble through the journey alone, if we shared nothing? It turns out, something amazing happened in my little life, and I am blessed by some pretty incredible love everywhere I go, so I want to tell you about this. I want to give you a little of my hope. Are you ready? Here we go.

I am a super heroine in my spare time. I leap tall buildings in a single bound just to find the best spot from which to watch the sunset. I support my local coffee shops. I make ten-minute rice in seven minutes (but I'm not one of those uncooked rice

people), and can Texas two-step in one step.

Spring 1994

When I was seventeen, I was totally pumped by the prospect of a new life at North Dakota State University. I was packed early (like, two months prior to the move date). My speech team friends helped me wash my car. Then, they covered it in shaving cream, just to show me their adoration. It did smell awfully nice. They capped that off by including a sandwich bag of quarters for a carwash. These are seriously good friends. Don't get me wrong. They're human. They will trash your stuff, but they'll clean it up, too. It will probably smell like aloe when they're done, and will have conditioned the vinyl on your vehicle.

I didn't tell my speech friends that I saved the quarters for laundry in the dorm. My best friend's little sister washed the car.

My older brother was also graduating. We aren't twins, but there are certain circumstances in which one sibling will end up in the classroom of another sibling. Above all, it made the graduation party cheaper for Mom and Dad.

At this time, my dad was going to pursue his dream of a medical career, after all of his years working at the power plant. My family had two garage sales and a furniture auction that summer. As previously mentioned, I was packed to go to college two months ahead of time. I had to decide what I was keeping and what had to GO. The house was rented out, and the new renters would be arriving the day after I left Washburn. My friends had scheduled a going away party, and there would be cake.

Mom and Dad had already gone on to move into their apartment and begin their college experience at the Science School. My brothers, Jeremy and Travis, were with them. My job was to make sure all of the lights were off in the house and lock up. I had the extra key. My family went in one direction, while I went in another. Yes, my parents went to college at the same time my brother, Jeremy, and I did. I think that helped us all understand our college communities better at the time. The young feel like they may conquer the world.

CHAPTER TWO

When I got to North Dakota State University in Fargo, I fell into my "joiner" pattern and became involved in lots of fun extra-curricular activities. I had new people to meet! I perfected extra-curricular yoga at the collegiate level, let me tell you. I stretched my schedule every which way I could. I worked with residence hall government, planning events and making candy bags to stick in mailboxes for each hall resident's birthday. That way, I would get to know more people's names.

I traveled with the speech and debate team on the weekends, so I made friends at other schools, which was very natural for me, having had a successful speech career in junior high and high school. I worked at the school newspaper and I became acquainted with all the student government kids and the administrators. I figured the more I did around campus, the more I would learn. My major was Communications, so I might as well communicate, right?

I had a great time at school. I was busy. I was productive.

I was totally a "joiner." I did not know how to say NO, to anyone. I had to be in on everything, or else I feared I'd miss something fun or important. In high school, I was a cheerleader and drama queen, and never slept.

When I look at the daily planner from my senior year, in-between and betwixt all of the stickers and hearts, reminders of social studies assignments, and rough drafts of football posters, interspersed with speech tournaments, play practice, and my job at the pizza parlor, I get tired and ponder taking a nap.

Extra-curricular activities are like yoga. If you stretch your limits, who knows where it will take you.

In addition to the newspaper, I started working at the college radio station, because I had a big crush on a guy who worked there. Okay, so that isn't the whole story. KDSU was the next door down the hall from *The Spectrum* newspaper office in the Memorial Union, so it seemed to be the natural progression of my media career.

I learned I really loved radio, so after about a year of producing an evening news and jazz program called *Nightbeat*, I left the college radio station and began working at a Top 40 music-intensive radio station in town on the weekends, on the overnight shift. After a while, the intense schedule of school, two deadlines a week at the paper, three radio stations began to seem like it was wearing on me, just a little.

10/27/97
"I'm very tired and very busy and very frustrated. Scot thinks if I begin journaling I will understand myself better. Let's face it, my job as a college journalist is to write. Lately I've been thinking I may be depressed, though I'd hate admit that to myself or anyone else. Something is just- wrong. I mean, come on! I am the Happy Girl. I'm just so tired all the time. I don't want to go to school anymore. Mom and Dad called today. Dad was accepted into a Physician Assistant school in Texas. They leave in March, and they said I need to make some decisions about my future."

I was a senior at North Dakota State University. I began having these crazy headaches, and all of my friends and a counselor at school thought I was clinically depressed. Clinically? Really? Everything was exhausting. Surprising, for the girl who slept maybe two hours a night, and only then, because she had to get some use out of her Paris Sport Club pajamas. I mean really, I ran until I hit a brick wall, collapsed, got up and ran again.

In recent days, however, my energy was dwindling. It was like I had molasses running through my veins. There was a short time when even getting out of bed was tough. My friends were standing by me, but it's pretty safe to say, this was widening everyone's eyes. They still won't admit it today, but I wonder if they were starting to think they should go through my purse to look for drugs. I was not acting like myself at all.

In the busy, blustery college town of Fargo, N.D., they see lots of kids go berserk when they get close to graduation. Maybe their relationships break up, or they don't know what to do with their lives. I mean, really, what do YOU want to do with the rest of your life? Your 22-year-old self should not be alone in the driver's seat of that decision, without some seriously well-marked roads. It's a good argument for internships and post-grad schools, to draw out the decision-making process.

The easiest and most obvious answer to all of that seems to land anywhere on the spectrum of depression. Perhaps the counselors and doctors think if they feed kids some kind of drug, they'll just snap out of it. Remember, this was in the Nineties. In those days, antidepressants were not quite as common as they have become. Maybe the patient will think she's getting help and her anxiety will just dissipate. It happens to lots of people, but in my case, maybe not. Looking back now, I don't think antidepressants were the answer.

Well, they certainly weren't for me.I was edgy, nervous all of the time. But, for conditions that need to be dealt with in young adults who are going to face serious issues like bills, relationships and possible environmental changes very soon, like cross-country moves, there has to be a more positive, healthy way to create serotonin.

I would arrive at work early to hang out in the studio with the fella who did the wildly popular weeknight show. He was funny, he was smart, and he was incredibly talented and put on a terrific "theater of the mind" radio show.

Within a couple of months, the program director recognized our chemistry and, as things often go in radio, we soon became the morning show. Spending time with him gave me a lot of privileges, which can be dizzying for a somewhat overworked girl who already meets two newspaper deadlines a week. For two years, we went to lots of concerts, and we rode in limousines, because the owner of the limo company traded service for advertising on the station.

Two years are a long time in a college life. We drank, quite a bit and usually for free. Mind you, I had never drunk alcohol before. My grades plummeted, but my

Communications courses kept my GPA up. Somehow, I managed to maintain at the newspaper, and I credit my fellow writers for their dedication to the student community and the others in the office. Certainly, this was the pinnacle of my little life. I was nominated for Homecoming Queen two years. At this time, all of my professors kept reminding me and pushing me toward my dream of television news reporting. Being on the radio, I was comfortable with a microphone, and not so comfortable with the camera. Still, I interned with all the television news crews in town.

It was during this time that I began to notice I was having a hard time holding onto things with my left hand. Carrying the cameras or awkward cables for the TV station was not easy. I attributed this to being right-handed and continued on my merry way. I would shrug and tell everyone I just did not have the hair to be on TV. I wasn't blonde, and everyone knows if you're going to be an anchor, you have to "look like your market." Besides, my focus was lacking and I totally screwed up those two years' worth of Homecoming Queen Interviews.

Let's talk about that for a moment. I can usually talk to anyone, anywhere. I can kick off a sing-along in an elevator, on a city bus, or even on a ferry over the

Corinth Sea in Greece. It's the dramatic cheerleader in me. In later years, I would be known to strike up a band. Even a rock band in front of thousands on a hundred degree day.

But when I sat across the table from the panel of interviewers for Homecoming Queen, I clammed up. I worked on a daily morning show and I could not answer questions of six people whom I knew. I shudder to think what their reaction might have been, but it's all a blur now._

That same fall, I began getting really nervous about things. Out of nowhere, my heart would start pounding and I couldn't breathe. It was close to Halloween. I thought I was developing some kind of phobia of jack-o-lanterns, or the dark. I would jump and screech sporadically, and my body would go numb. I had spurts of confusion.

I made life pretty miserable, I think, for my boyfriend. He absolutely did not know what to make of all this. He thought it was a ploy for attention, and things between us got tense.

"You're no fun to be around when you act like this," he said. "Just look at yourself."

I couldn't see myself then. I couldn't see anything.

Imagine feeling like your air is being cut off, your heart is racing, and you are going to die. That's how it was, almost daily. I didn't want to be too dramatic.

I was out of contact with most of my friends because I needed to be with the guy all I could. If I spent time with other people, I usually felt better, more even-tempered and calm, but the boyfriend would get upset if I scarcely spoke with anyone else.

Girls: don't ever date or spend your time with someone like this. This was a fine line to walk, due to my responsibilities as an editor of the college newspaper, and talking to college students, faculty, and administration was my whole existence. It was how I was getting paid, and that was how I was gaining the experience to become the newswoman I planned to be. Eventually, to avoid the uncomfortable situations, he won.

My head hurt. Maybe it was stress. I was grasping for something familiar, and I thought he was it, because sometimes he was in the mood to be my rescuer and help me keep breathing through what we thought were those crazy panic attacks, when one side of my body would go numb and my vision would get blurry. I would become very afraid when I couldn't breathe and my legs would wobble out from under me, all while maintaining consciousness. Most of the time, he wasn't in the mood for this bad behavior, poor guy. He told me to just stop it.

1/11/1998

In January of my senior year at school, I had a dream opportunity: I was offered an internship at a network news bureau in Washington, D.C.!

Steve Sando was legendary at North Dakota State. He had worked at KDSU and had once been an editor of our college paper, *The Spectrum,* years before I'd ever hung my trench coat on the door. He had been me when he was my age. Now he was Director of Technical Operations for CBS (say that three times fast!), Washington Bureau. I was dying to talk to him about how he had made that jump.

The very classy Karen Severtsen, Director of Programming at KDSU, had known Steve since his college days and gave me his phone number. I took a deep breath, set my notebook at 90 degrees on my desk, and dialed. I learned all of the stories were also true about Steve being an exceptional guy, as well.

During my interview with this man, he very coolly

offered me an internship with Dan Rather, CBS This Morning, and Face The Nation. Like, in Washington, D.C. I asked him to repeat himself, although I was writing down every word he said.

Did he just give me my big break? I had wanted to work in television news since my dad was in Desert Storm, when the only channel we ever watched at our house was the news. I peered over Wolf Blitzer's shoulder, looking to catch a glimpse of my dad in the Arabian Desert. I saw Richard Jaco ducking when the missiles flew overhead, and Scud Stud Arthur Kent's photocopied headshot hung in our yearbook staff office of my high school. I felt that doing the news was one way I could serve my country. My dreams were all going to happen now. I was going to do *the news*. Despite this being everything I ever dreamed of, I remember not wanting to get on the plane. The morning we were driving into Minneapolis-St. Paul International Airport, my heart began to pound. I had that terrifying rollercoaster feeling.

"No, no, no," I said to my boyfriend, quietly pressing my feet against the floor of his car, trying to hit the imaginary brakes.

"Not yet. I can't do it yet."

As if the plane would wait until I calmed down.

"Just remember I am so proud of you," he said. "Be good."

Of course I would be good. I only knew how to be good. It would be great. I always work hard, and if I know someone is counting on me, I work harder.

As soon as I got into my room at the women's dorm in D.C. where a lot of interns stayed, I called home and spoke to my parents.

"Can I come home now?" I asked quietly, knowing I shouldn't be voicing my dissatisfaction or worries. I felt the smallness of my five-by-eight room and the bigness of the city, as a Midwestern girl who wasn't sure she was ready for this, and there was a clanging in my head.

"It's a little too late for that," Dad said, reminding me I had just moved out of my apartment, crossed the country in an airplane, and was now signed up for fifteen credits of experiential intern learning this semester.

"You'll feel better in the morning." I decided he was right, and he handed the phone to Mom. She told me to make my room homey and get some rest. I made my little dorm room as "homey" as possible with what I had rolled into my duffle bag: a Winnie-the-Pooh pillow case, my lighthouse blanket, an alarm clock, and one stuffed lion. Mom and Dad had given me Dr. Seuss' "Oh The Places You Will Go!" for Christmas, so I managed to pack around that, as well. In those days, packing for the airplane was not nearly what it is today. I was able to bring my full-size shampoo, conditioner, and enough beauty products for a three-month television internship.

My friend Heather had gone out to D.C. with me. She arranged a congressional internship so I wouldn't have to do this three-month trip alone. I think Heather, having seen my personality change and my confidence drop over the previous two years, was nervous to allow me out of her sight and across the country! I have good friends. After dropping off our stuff at the dorm, and making our calls home, our NDSU friend Ana picked us up and took us to Starbucks.

Being a Midwesterner, it was my first trip to a Starbucks, of which we'd only heard fairy tales. The coffee movement had not yet reached its pinnacle back home. Although, as a good French-Greek-German girl, I've been guzzling java juice since pre-K, and I had no idea how pivotal this night and the coffee outing would be on my future pocketbook. There we were, three hip college chicks, living it up at Starbucks in Washington, D.C. in the Nineties.

We had the world by the tail. They make movies about this stuff.

I didn't feel better in the morning, as Dad had suggested, or the day after that. I had a countdown written out. I set my tray with my quartered grapefruit and coffee down on the pink cloth at the breakfast table where Heather was seated alone and dropped myself into the chair next to her.

"Ninety-four days until I go home," I sighed. "Ninety-four days…"

"Don't *do* that," Heather said, over a dormitory breakfast of pears and cornflakes. She did not look forward to my daily countdown announcement.

"Try to enjoy it." Given my media experience, this is exactly what I should have been doing at exactly the right time. But something didn't feel right, and that something was a little numbness here and there and thunder banging headaches. It was going to be tough to be impressive. I would have to fake a lot.

I slept with my light on at the end of my bed in my small "cell" in the intern dorm on Capitol Hill, if I slept at all. It was pretty tiny. I am claustrophobic, and had a phobia of cockroaches, having never seen one.

This anxiety felt much like my jack-o-lantern phobia back home. Now I don't know into what state I would have escalated myself had I actually laid eyes on a bug, but at that time, there were no such terrors. A small town girl, fearing bugs and big cities, with pounding in her skull and numbness creeping in on one side of her body was not a happy soul in that little room. I prayed.

Job 11:16-19 "You will forget your misery; you will remember it as waters that have passed away. And your life will be brighter than the noonday; its darkness will be like the morning. And you will have confidence, because there is hope; you will be protected and take your rest in safety. You will lie down, and none will make you afraid; many will entreat your favor."

CHAPTER THREE

Walking into CBS, I could hear the Rocky Theme
playing. Wait. No, maybe that was the Mary Tyler
Moore Theme. At any rate, once I survived the
terrifying ascent of the incredibly long DuPont Circle
escalator out of the Metro, and learned about myself
that I don't care for heights, I walked down the block
feeling like I could pretty much conquer anything.

I mean, seriously. I was spending my days at the nerve
center of CBS News. Let me just tell you that, while big
and important, any journalist anywhere, who broadcasts
a story – via television, radio, newspaper or on the
internet – and reaches an audience, has just as big of a
responsibility in their message whether they are at the
CBS Bureau in Washington, D.C., or the KDSU
Newsroom, on the campus of North Dakota State
University.

Other soap operas were playing themselves out in our
nation's capital. The Monica Lewinsky scandal broke
and things were very strained in Washington. The
network's intern coordinator, Jackie, was not as

friendly as I'd imagined, or as nice as she had portrayed herself on the phone. Because I had walked into this opportunity rather gingerly, I think she had it in her mind that I was "one of those interns." I was not.

The morning that story broke, as I walked from one end of the CBS newsroom to the other to get a foot-high stack of newspapers off of a desk, which was just part of my job. I had a vague awareness of a bright light off to my left, and flipped my hair over. My mother, watching the morning news from North Dakota, and no doubt whispering to herself something about atrocities in the highest office in our nation, while praying for the future of our country, noticed a familiar hair-flipping in the back, over Dan Rather's left shoulder. She set her coffee down and crawled across the living room floor, exclaiming,

"That's my baby girl!" just as I was making my return trip across that huge room. I didn't set out to do it that morning, but I accidentally accomplished one of my life's goals: to appear on national morning television. My mother saw me! That counts.

Not so long after that, I ran into Dan Rather in the hallway. Being my cheerleader self, who suffers from no real social anxiety whatsoever, I greeted him. He asked what school I attended. Naturally, being a Texan, he was very polite to me. When the story got back to

24

Intern Coordinator Jackie, it was that I had sauntered right up and elbowed his security detail out of the way. Jackie informed me, in no uncertain terms, that my internship was over and I was going back to Fargo.

The head honcho, our NDSU friend Steve, took me out to lunch and said I didn't have to leave, that I had done nothing wrong, but I foresaw nothing but problems with an already miffed intern coordinator, so I made the decision to go home. There was plenty waiting for me there, including the buildup to graduation.

"Go home and do radio, kid," Steve advised me. "Have fun."

"Life is so interesting," said Karen, my mentor back at the college radio station in Fargo. "That's why we bother to get out of bed in the morning - just to see what's going to happen."

I returned to North Dakota, having lost forty pounds in the month I was away. I believed to my very core that I had failed and would never amount to anything. I felt completely defeated, and as though all that I'd worked to build all my life to that point had come crashing down. My Girl Scout troop toured a TV/radio station in sixth grade; I set my sights on being a newswoman and that was *that*. I thought I disappointed everyone who had ever believed in me. I took comfort in the radio station I had called home. I needed to rack up more internship hours doing *something,* somewhere, so I could graduate in May.

 Shortly after my arrival home, my boyfriend and I broke up. He was dating someone else at the station, and on the air, in front of our whole listenership, regarded me as a "depressed psychotic." To the entire listening area! *Halloo!* He would taunt me every day with statements like, "Everybody sees what's wrong with you, but you."

We had a lack of communication. I had an agreement to finish up my intern hours at the station, so I did a lot of commercial production that spring.

It was painful and ugly. Headaches and panic attacks were almost constant which means the feeling of numbness was overtaking my left arm and leg and the left side of my face. I was gasping for air when this happened, It was so weird, and I thought it was just because I was so worked up and could not keep food down. Not a pretty time. My then ex-boyfriend demanded again I stop with the ploys for attention.

3/25/98

My ex-boyfriend asked me if I'd like to go out to dinner

for my birthday. I jumped at the chance for something familiar. I think it was Maya Angelou who said, "When people show you who they are, you should believe them." It was a bad idea to go out and spend time with him and expect it to go well. I turned down an evening with a plethora of my friends to have dinner with him.

We went to the Greek restaurant, which I loved. We fought; I don't remember what caused it. What is it ever about? At what I determined the end of the fight, I ran through some icy alleyways back to my apartment. He chased me, and because he has longer legs, caught me. A police car pulled up, seemingly out of nowhere. It is a well-patrolled neighborhood. The cop was probably thinking I was being beaten or manhandled by this creep. He ended up dragging me in to the emergency room, and I had a psychological evaluation. I remember being very annoyed with him.

Through staff changes at the radio station, he was now the program director, and therefore in charge of writing a letter to my communication department advisor at school, saying that yes, I had completed "X" number of weekly intern hours at the station, so I could graduate from the university in less than two months. My ex-boyfriend was my supervisor. And he was flaunting a new girlfriend. And I was unsure of my direction in life. The psychologist in the emergency room had no problem seeing why this was all stressful. Nope, it's all good.

"She's very good at saying that everything is fine in a very light way."

Yes, I was screaming inside. *I am the happy girl. Ask anyone! I'm a great actress. Won an acting scholarship. And it's my birthday.*

I remember thinking during one anxious episode that I didn't *have* to be so riled up. But I felt like I couldn't stop, as though I would die. I couldn't breathe and I was numb and afraid. The room was spinning and I didn't understand why. I couldn't find a shred of the normalcy and "old me" that I longed for. I couldn't find any of that person. I *missed* me. At this time, I felt like a total loser. *I* was not supposed to have these worries. Not *me*. I was one of those kids who live by her daily planner. I felt like nothing, at what I had thought would be a really exciting time in my life. When did it get so off track? I had done everything right.

'I think I have a brain tumor," I said to Heather one day that spring. We were walking past the fountains on campus, and I was thankful she had returned from her internship. "Something's going on. My mom thinks I have a brain tumor or that I'm on drugs."

'No," Heather's eyes got wide and she nearly choked.

28

"That's NOT funny. Don't say things like that. It'll be okay. Just give it time."

With that, we went to the coffee cart in the Memorial Union to get a latte`. The caffeine always seemed to make the headaches go away. I told everyone I was just addicted to caffeine. Everyone was. It was the "in" addiction. That explained why I had such piercing headaches if I didn't drink any coffee or soda in the morning, right? But nobody else seemed to get the sudden headaches like I did. My headaches were famous.

I was scared and I was miserable, and *so* emotionally fragile. I would be driving, singing along with the radio, and the left side of my body would go numb instantly. I got very disoriented and very confused. This happened many times, and I would pull over to the side of the road, or just keep driving, until I could remember where I was going and what to do when I got there. After one of those episodes, the day would be shot. I had very little ability to concentrate, and an even smaller sense of purpose. I thought I was going completely off the deep end.

I did not want them to be right about me being depressed. I did not want to feel marred or damaged in any way. I also did not want anyone to know about it. All of my friends were so excited about graduation. I did not want to worry them. I didn't want to stress anyone out. I didn't want to be the downer, because I was accustomed to planning our social activities, being the Radio Girl. This was getting weird.

CHAPTER FOUR

My dad was beginning his medical school in San Antonio, TX. He was already there. Mom, my brother Travis and I were still in North Dakota, planning to move to Texas when I managed to graduate from college and Travis' school year was completed in May.

"Come to Texas and lie by the pool for a few weeks," my mom said. "You don't have to find a job right away."

TEXAS? Isn't Texas just one big desert? I don't know anyone in Texas! That would ruin my social life! What would I ever do in Texas?

I walked the stage at the Fargodome, proud that I had gotten my Mass and Speech Communications double major finished in a mere four years.

The week of graduation, I called the University President's office to get permission to decorate my mortarboard. College graduates all over the country do this every year, but it takes a special kind of nerd to get permission from Administration. We'd heard you could get in trouble for it.

A couple of my best Blue Key National Honor Fraternity buddies, Carl and John, gathered with me, glue and glitter, to get this mission accomplished. When we were finished, John had the symbol of his fraternity on his cap. Carl would be sporting an NDSU-friendly theme on his head, and I had a winking smiley face atop my noggin, in a blue glitter that would match my Blue Key Honor cord. I still have it, all these years later.

There are experiences in the mind that are as clear as if they had occurred five minutes ago. Especially for women, as we recall our very best hair days. Who doesn't look tanned and tone, at twenty-two? As we were milling about behind the stage at the Fargodome, a woman none of us had ever seen came up behind me and ripped my mortarboard off of my head, bobby pins flying everywhere. My eyes flew out of my head and bounced across the Fargodome parking lot as I exclaimed, "Whoa! HAIR!"

The university photographer, Dan Koeck, was taking pictures, as the aforementioned nameless woman barely looked at me and told me more than asked, "Wanna go change your cap."

"Excuse me," I altered my Spectrum News Editor /
Radio News, perhaps slightly condescending Delivery
Tone. "No ma'am. I called President Plough's office. I
have permission for this mortarboard. My mom has
traveled across the country. How will she see me from
up in the seats if not for this cap?"

I stood, in shock and lidless, as said nameless woman
marched off with my cap to corroborate that I had
permission to wear a smiley face on my head so my
mom could see me from up in the seats while I crossed
the stage to receive my degree. All I could do was try to
smooth out my hair, and gather the bobby pins. How
rude.

Meanwhile, Carl and John were reminding me to
breathe. It's okay; I'm not a crier. There were some
guys we didn't know who had somehow managed to fly
in under the radar with beer logos on their caps. Jerks.
I'm just the one who got caught. That's what always
keeps me out of trouble. If anyone had gotten caught, it
would have been me. Therefore, I wasn't going to
attempt any trouble. Carl picked up the rest of my
bobby pins and handed them to me. I squared my
shoulders, walked back to the door where the
mortarboard thief stood talking to President Plough's
administrative assistant, Stephanie. She turned and
handed me my cap back, without a word. I went to the

ladies' room and fixed my hair.

I begrudgingly took Mom up on the invitation to follow them to San Antonio. What else was I going to do at that point?
My friends were all headed in different directions, and with all of the stress the last few years, it was clear I needed to clear my head before I found my direction, too.

Upon arriving in Texas, "a whole 'nuther country," I spent a couple of weeks lying by the pool and drinking iced tea, just as Mom had suggested. Maybe the sunshine helped, with its Vitamin D.

One day, driving past a taco restaurant, I saw a radio remote broadcast in action. The radio station's van was painted with a huge, bright logo, and the mast shot up, clear to the stratosphere. I was excited at the prospect of radio people, and I stopped. I walked over to the booth and asked the group if they needed any weekenders.

"Do we! We always need talented people! Got any experience?" asked the smiling woman with the microphone. I reflected on a year at the college radio station and two years' worth of morning radio in Fargo, and, holding up my thumb and index finger, told her, oh, I had a little experience.

"Great! Got a tape?" Still smiling, Diane Travis asked me. She was flanked by three promotions crewmembers, like she was a movie star.

I whipped a cassette out of my purse that had been meticulously labeled with my name, website (thanks to my genius brother), e-mail and telephone number.

The next day, her boss called me and offered me a dinner interview, after which I got a tour of the coolest radio station I had ever seen. It was six floors into the sky, with huge windows that overlooked the highways and byways of San Antonio. During this tour, KSMG Program Director Andy Holt offered me a full-time job doing seven to midnight, including the Awesome 80s at 8 show. In contrast to my part-time radio gigs in Fargo, I would have a salary, medical insurance, life insurance, and a retirement plan. I fell in with a group of really wonderful co-workers, and I told everyone back home it was surely God's Will. It was definitely more than luck. I was going to be the fun, awesome Night Girl on the Radio.

I am never going to worry about anything again. God's got me.

I got an apartment with a pool outside my door. I bought furniture. I loved having a grownup paycheck and feeling like I was well on my way to bigger and better things. I loved the Texas sunshine. Maybe the "depression" I had experienced in Fargo was just a touch of Seasonal Affected Disorder.

Still, especially at night, after my show at midnight, I had occasional and intense bouts of anxiety and numbness. Maybe they were right back at school. Maybe I was depressed. Maybe I had a hard time calming down at midnight, after being "keyed-up" on-air all evening. Maybe I had to give it time, and it would get better eventually. Occasional headaches and numb panic attacks were better than the constant ones I had in Fargo.

See, I'd tell myself. *I'm already feeling better.*

I made friends. Life got easier and I thought I was really making progress. I was hostessing party buses to Austin concerts and bringing bands onstage. I did dance parties on the Riverwalk almost every Friday night. I was having a blast!

Then I began getting sick. This was different than it had been in Fargo. It wasn't just shortness-of-breath and numbness attacks. This was sick.

Due to my evening work schedule, I was able to accompany Mom as we explored San Antonio during the days. I tired easily. My headaches got worse, much more severe than they had ever been in college. Every couple of weeks, I would have flu-like symptoms that would knock my socks off, with violent vomiting. I couldn't even believe how sick I was, the vomiting seemed so animated in its fountainous nature. Sometimes I wasn't able to move, I was so sick.

"Migraines," I was told. "Tension headaches."

"Oh, you're just sick," said one nurse at an urgent care clinic.

That much I knew. The pain in my neck was becoming intense. I wondered *why* I was so sick. During one of these visits, a doctor told me, "I would say possible viral meningitis, but if you're still able to walk around, you must be fine."

Therefore, on the days when I was so ill I couldn't move, I looked like I was just being stubborn and lazy. I had no excuses.

Something is wrong in my head. If I'm "depressed," then it's just a chemical imbalance, like they say. How do I fix that? I want this to be over.

A chemical imbalance sounded less dramatic than the fear. My ability to manage my checkbook was dwindling. I got confused figuring simple addition and subtraction. I moved back in with my parents to avoid money problems. One morning, my mother heard a loud crash from the bathroom. I had passed out in the shower. At that point, I had not felt well for weeks. My parents were annoyed with me, because they thought I had been slipped some kind of drug in a drink at a bar the night before. Well, okay, that time I probably had been slipped something in a drink at a bar, sent to me by a stranger. Thank God for surrounding me with my faithful promotions crew, who acted as best friends and bodyguards. They removed the beverage as I took one sip, and didn't let me out of their sight as we left and they dropped me at home.

I promised my parents I would be more responsible.

Summer 1999

The time came for my family to go north again, but only as far as Copperas Cove, Texas, near Fort Hood. Dad had another year of school. I had a job and friends and I was doing okay, so I stayed in San Antonio, working at my radio station and happily housesitting for some wonderful family friends, Grammy and Grampy Baker, for the summer. We had a shakeup at the station, and I spent that summer co-hosting The Sonny Melendrez and Company morning show. Sonny is one of those exhilarated individuals who make you feel like paying it forward, helping an old lady across the street, and teaching the world to sing, all in the same day. Being both a morning person and a night person, I enjoyed being back on morning radio and working with my friends, but as summer wore on, my 80s show called to me from the other side of the clock.

It was baffling to me how weak I had become, but the panic attacks were rare at that point. I had lost some weight, and was glad about that, in the sort of way you might be glad about something you have achieved at a cost.

At the end of the summer, I moved into another house with two friends, Brent and Del Mar. I thought it would be fun to have housemates, like on MTV's Real World. At this point, I was thankful I was back to doing my show alone at night, so no one could watch me drop my head on the counter after each twenty-second break.

"MAGIC 105.3...IT'S THE 80'S AT 8 WITH JOSIE BLAINE... THAT'S NOT AN APPLIANCE, IT'S MY NAME...YOUR REQUESTS AT 470-KSMG... OMD... IF YOU LEAVE...ON MAGIC."

KONK! The coolness of the console countered the heat in my flushed face. Oh my goodness, that had taken every ounce of everything I had, but I would muster up enough strength to be able to do it again in a few minutes. I was never too sick to be a radio star! I always loved my job so much that I didn't like to take a vacation or a day off due to sickness, even when the headaches were bad. If I could stand up, I would be standing up behind a microphone.

My neck hurt. My chiropractor kept trying to adjust my C-2, which is one of the cervical bones in the neck. My neck hurt all the time and I was constantly dizzy. Somehow, I was still functioning. If you smile enough, people just think your elevator doesn't go all the way to the top. Playing the friendly, smart ditz works for a while. I don't think anyone knew how much of my body I couldn't feel.

At this point, I noticed that I was getting even weaker on the left side of my body. It wasn't just becoming numb sometimes. It was a weird numb all the time, like when your leg is asleep and right before it wakes up, there's that horrific pins and needles feeling? Welcome to my left side.

I tried to do little things, like hold the phone with my left hand. It was very difficult, but I didn't mention it to anybody, because I was embarrassed to seem like some kind of wimp. I thought I had become too dependent on my right hand, so I made a conscious effort to use the left one. I just did more push-ups against the counter console in the studio during my show. My feeling didn't return.

The end of August came. It was time to take Travis back to North Dakota and settle him into a residence hall at North Dakota State University, where I had attended college. I think I was more excited than he. Though I had really *hoped* he'd choose my alma mater and be a Bison, I didn't pressure him. Much. I did, however, do all the right Big Sister Things, like buy him Green Stuff for graduation.

I woke up on a Saturday morning, while it was still dark, and began the journey up to Fort Hood, to pick up my mom and brother. I was in unbelievable pain the whole way. I pulled over to rest twice, and doubled back a few times in the darkness to make sure I was on the right highway. I probably drove the same ten-mile stretch of highway 281 three times. I just couldn't remember where I was and I couldn't see very well. My car was floating along on angels' wings, because there is no way I drove three hours feeling as I did.

I finally got to my parents' place as the sun was rising. We packed all of Travis' things in my car and settled in for the long haul. Near Waco, Mom decided to take the wheel. "Are you aware that you're not keeping the car in your lane?" she asked.

"Mo*ther*, I haven't been *aware* of anything for a really long time."

I slept in the backseat of my own car as Mom and Travis shared the rest of the driving.

The next day, we stopped for lunch near Omaha, NE. Ever so calmly after eating, I walked into the ladies' room and got sick. Projectile vomiting a` la Linda Blair is the best way to describe it. And I had drunk lots of lemonade at lunch. I would guess I hurled a bright yellow fountain of lemonade about six feet across the floor. I splashed cold water on my face as an unsuspecting Nebraskan entered the ladies' room. I slipped out quietly, not making eye contact. Just as calmly, I rejoined my mom and brother at the table.

"I just threw up," I announced brightly, but so as not to call attention to our table.

I don't think they thought much of it at the time. They were discussing something and pretty much ignored my unpleasant statement. I was always getting sick. At this point, I'll bet they thought I was bulimic or something.

In North Dakota, it became necessary to pay a visit to the chiropractor. Dr, Alisa had attended to my chiropractic considerations in college. We got Travis settled at NDSU.

By the time we got to western North Dakota to see relatives, I was sleeping twenty hours a day. I'm sure to the outsider; I looked like a typical young adult who slept all of the time. But my family and friends knew something was serious now, because with my usual energy level and my usual body clock, this was not normal. I had to take a hefty dose of my Aunt Bonnie's migraine medicine in order to sit at the dinner table with the family one night. It was worth it.

Nothing beats a steak at Aunt Bonnie and Uncle Leonard's farm in North Dakota.

In the morning, when Bonnie was pouring coffee, I held up my empty cup. It shook. It nearly shook out of my hand. Mom, Bonnie and I looked at my hand, and they looked at me. That had never happened before. None of us knew what to say. I set the cup down and Bonnie filled it.

CHAPTER FIVE

After breakfast, Mom and I went to the mall. I followed her into a store.

She heard, "Clomp. Sliiiiide. Clomp. Sliiiiide." My left foot was having a hard time keeping up, and my sandal was dragging with every step.

"What is *that?*" My mother's eyes were the size of Greek dinner plates as she whipped around and demanded to know if that was a new dance move.

"Sometimes my left foot drags a little." Boy, this was embarrassing. I didn't want her to notice. As a completely capable, very busy young woman, with several jobs I'd just finished at the end of college, suddenly my weaknesses were piling up on me. I thought I did okay at work at the radio station. This hadn't happened before.

My mother drove the entire trip back to Texas. She

suggested that maybe I had Multiple Sclerosis, because of the shaking and the dragging. We talked about what an MS diagnosis would mean, and Mom said that with the right medication, I could lead a virtually symptom-free life. My friend Heather had MS, and was doing great with it.

It was very sobering to think of having something actually "wrong" with me, but I, too, was getting to the point that I just wanted to know *why* I was going out of my mind and why my neck and head hurt with numbness in my leg all the time.

I dropped Mom off in Copperas Cove, and somehow got myself back down to San Antonio. Traffic must have been light. This was the 29th of August. I went on the air that night, and the next day, managed to squeeze in an appointment with my doctor. I kept trying to tell her about this awful ache in the back of my head and neck.

"Does the pain go away when you lie down?" she asked.

"Sometimes."

"It's probably just a pinched nerve or something. Go home and lie down."

I did my show that night as well.

"Oh, I think I'm going to die," I told Tom when I walked in the door that afternoon. "My mom thinks I have a brain tumor."

"It's not a too-mah," he said, doing his best Arnold Schwarzenegger impression, from Kindergarten Cop.

I made it through my show, with no problems during the 80s at 8.

The next day, I awoke around noon, with something new. I couldn't tolerate standing, sitting or lying down. My neck hurt so badly I really just wanted to chop my own head off to relieve some of the pressure. It felt like my head would explode. I did what a lot of people do when they're sick. I called my mommy.

"My neck hurts. I can't do anything. It just hurts," I sobbed into the phone, being very much a baby. I'm not used to crying, so this was a little strange for both of us.

"Your C-2 must be way out of whack. See if you can get in to see Dr. Fielden," Mom offered.

I have no idea how I got there. I drove about five minutes to the chiropractor's office in an almost unconscious state. I am very sorry to the other people driving on the road that day. Monica was the only one in the office when I arrived. She informed me that Dr. Fielden was at lunch.

"Sorry, Josie. He'll be back at three."

I looked at the clock. One thirty. How would I get back home and then return to the office in an hour?

"Can I just wait here?"

She said of course, sure, that would be no problem, and must have sensed how very much an emergency my visit was. She walked to the back and had Dr. Fielden with her when she returned.

Dr. Fielden is a congenial practitioner. He's friendly and has a great manner about him. We had a jovial doctor-patient relationship, so when the mood was very dark, he got right down to business on my skeleton. He something was definitely cutting off blood flow to my head, and that my face looked gray. If it felt no better the next day, I was to come back.

I went home and almost overslept for my show. I got to the station by six, recorded a few commercials into the computer system in the production department, decided to finish the dubs later and stopped to chat with the creative services director, my good friend Ric.

"You don't look so good," Ric said, waving his hand in front of my face.

"Oh gee, thanks," said I, staring into space, not seeing his hand.

"You'd better go talk to Andy. See if he'll let you go home."

"Okay," I shrugged.

In a trance, I wobbled down the hall, bouncing from wall to wall, to my program director's office. He wasn't very pleased. It was 6:10. My show started at seven and I had to be in the studio at 6:45.

He called out to Tom in the next office.

"Tom? Can you cover her show?"

"I've got my kids tonight, Andy," Tom hollered back.

Pain and guilt were simultaneously tearing me apart.

"You know I can do it every night," I told him.
"Tonight, I can't." Andy dismissed me without another

word.

Upon my arrival at the house, I tried lying in my bed. Too uncomfortable. Neck pain. I had to physically hold onto the back of my neck if I was sitting, standing, or lying down. My room was too small and the walls seemed to be closing in on me. The ceiling fan looked like it was going to fall at any moment.

I migrated to the living room. I felt like Goldilocks. I couldn't find a spot that was "just right." I turned on the television for company, but it was too loud. If I turned it off, the house was too quiet. My housemates were not home. I couldn't lie still, and was writhing in pain. I felt like I was being strangled to death, and I couldn't get a single breath of air. I called my mom every ten minutes.

"I'm so sick, Mom."

Mom, being a few hours north, recommended I call Taylor to come and sit with me.

It's truly a blessing to have friends who would do anything for you at the drop of a hat, in the twinkling of an eye. I have many such friends. Taylor, one of my best buddies from the Magic promotions crew, was sitting at my feet within moments. The crew takes good care of the air talent. They make sure we look good, get to the right place on time, we have everything we need, never get thirsty, are never accosted by stalkers, and generally are our lifeblood. During one of my many phone calls to my mother, she asked to speak with Taylor. I could barely speak just then for all the pain, so I was in an almost-crying state. I never cry. I am not a moaner.

Holding that back was tough for me, because it felt like my head had perhaps been hit very hard, or was being twisted off. What had I done to get myself into this situation? I thought, *if this is how I'm going to die, come on! How much worse can it possibly get?*

"Please take her in to the emergency room," Mom pleaded with Taylor on one of my frequent phone calls. "This has been going on for years. We have to get to the bottom of this once and for all."

 Normally, I would have declined, saying no, I would be fine after some sleep. However, I knew I wasn't going to get any rest and decided if I was going to die that night, it might as well be in a hospital, where they are prepared for such things, and not where my roommates would come home and find a dead *me* in the living room. Neither Taylor nor I knew where the hospital was. Then I arrived upon a brilliant idea, amidst the death grip pain had on the upper part of my body.

"I know! We can follow the blue and white "H" hospital signs!" Like it was a new idea. How clever of the sign people to put those things up here and there.

Taylor guided me out to his tiny car, and, blindly, off we went. Neither of us was sure where we would find a hospital. A brilliant light bulb flashed above my head.

The road was bumpy. I vomited out the passenger door of the car during most of the trip. Lemonade again. It was the only thing I could stand all day. Taylor, bless his heart, grabbed a Jimmy Buffet t-shirt from one of his Jimmy Buffet college fraternity events off the floorboards in the back seat so I could wipe off my face.

"Oh, Taylor, this…isn't very… ladylike," I mourned.

"I've seen you be ladylike," he replied. "Now let's get you well. I don't like Jimmy Buffet anyway."

The car stopped short outside the Northeast Baptist Emergency Room. We shuffled inside, and I dropped my purse on the desk, causing a perfectly friendly person to jump and whip around in her seat.

"Can I help you?" asked a smiling, blue-eyed face from behind the counter.

"Yes, I'm... sick."

Two large bodies were on either side of me, and I was taken to some curtained-off area within the ER. Not long after, I was given a shot of something to reduce swelling. The chart says Demerol. I was breathing again.

Soon, Taylor was sitting next to me in an exam room, holding my hand, and I had traded my San Antonio Spurs Championship t-shirt and shorts for a hospital gown, with a sheet to cover up with. The Demerol was beginning to make me more comfortable. It was working. Very well.

The events from then on are something of a blur. I see scenes, bits and pieces.

The young PA on duty rushed in, glanced at me and said to the room, "Okay, we're going to do a CT scan."

Now, somewhere in the back of my humble, financially responsible, North Dakota brain, I could hear myself thinking, "CT scans are EXPENSIVE. But I have insurance now. I have a JOB."

And they wheeled me off.

Now, listen. I am *way* claustrophobic. I think it stems from the torture of being trapped inside a green Holly Hobby sleeping bag when I was five, with all holes blocked off. My big brother viewed seriously his role to toughen me up for the world. However, combined with my drug-induced sleepiness and the fact that they only put you halfway in the tube for a CT scan, I was fine.

Later, PA Larry Tatum is shuffling papers, bending down and looking very carefully into my eyes, telling me, "You're going to have to be hospitalized. Your CT scan came back...abnormal."

"Drugged up" is the best descriptive I can give you. I can still see his eyes, and he was much more concerned about it than I was at that moment. For all the "feel better" injections they had already given me, I mustered up my best "drunk-acting-sober" face and looked back at him just as carefully.

"Okay. Taylor, call my mom." My good friend, who was also hearing this crazy news, unfiltered, had my cell phone. I handed him the responsibility of relaying it to my parents.

Taylor called my parents. Then Larry Tatum called my parents. I'm not altogether sure what those conversations were like, I just know I was really sleepy and didn't want Taylor to leave. He sat next to me and held my hand.

Every five minutes or so I would ask, "How long now? Is my mom here yet?"

"They'll be here in about two hours."

Finally at about four a.m., Mom rushed into the room, Dad behind her. I just *knew* when I'd finally see her; she'd be wearing a Texas t-shirt. Her face was as white as a sheet. Why do people say, "…white as a sheet?" Maybe the sheets weren't white. Mom's face was as white as snow on a dark night. Dad was gray with worry.

"Mom!" I exclaimed gleefully. "I have a *brain*! They took pictures of it!"

For a long time, through my college years, and especially in the past few months, Mom had thought I was completely ditzy, possibly on drugs, and certainly not myself.

"I know," she said. "Hush, it's okay, baby girl. I love you."

I remember my feet were cold. Dad, the curious medical professional that he is, knew exactly where to go to get me a pair of those little booties that hospitals issue patients, with the "sergeant stripes" grips on the bottoms. He either got them from the nurses' station, or he went through enough cabinets and drawers to find something to cover my feet, because my toes were turning as blue as my indigo toenail polish.

They finally put me in a hospital room, blocked it off as private, and brought in recliners, pillows and blankets for my parents. Sweet, patient Taylor, who had to work later that morning, went home to catch some shut-eye. What a good friend.

So what does "abnormal" mean on a CT scan? Nobody seemed to have an answer. At least not an answer I would hear. Whatever the answer was, it kind of all made sense—the headaches for the last few years, the irrational fights with my mom and my boyfriend, the lack of concentration in school but hyper focus at work (or maybe that was just my left brain taking over). I remember one Communication Analysis Group assignment, during which I absolutely could not, to save my life, connect in my mind the meaning of the word, "implications." I passed that class with a B. Looking at my college transcript today, it is painfully obvious to me when the problem began.

The next thing I can recall is that it was morning, and a neurosurgeon was coming in at 9:30. Everyone still seemed to be in a panic around me, but trying really hard to smile and be sweet.

What? Why is everyone freaked out? Do I have a brain tumor or something?

I was mostly being facetious. Whaddya know? As it turned out, I *did* have a brain tumor. I had a radio show. I had friends. I had a life. I had magnolias blooming outside my door. I had a brain tumor. Well, didn't that just beat all? Now what?

Humph. I guess that explains a few things. Wait until I tell Heather. Ok, who's going to fix me?

It was a big mass, and evidently in a hard place in which to operate, wrapped around my brain stem, where heart and lung functions operate. If they didn't pick me up and take me to the brain surgeon in Phoenix, *stat*, it kind of looked like I wouldn't see Labor Day. Today is Thursday. Decisions. In a hurry. He suggested our best option was a surgeon in Phoenix, but he didn't think there was time to get me there.

"There *is* a new guy over at University Hospital who does this kind of surgery, but he's extremely busy," Dr. Garza-Vale shared with my parents. My dad thought there would be no harm in calling anyway, because there was no time to waste.

Dr. Garza-Vale called Dr. Christopher Bogaev's office.

Instead of a nurse, or a secretary, Dr. Bogaev answered.

"Send her over here," Dr. Bogaev told him. He had just moved his family into a new house and it wasn't organized yet. He probably had plans that involved their patio and grill that weekend, but he agreed to give up his holiday weekend to save *my* life. Wow. After hanging up the phone, Dr. Bogaev called his nurse Cindy.

"There's a 23-year-old girl at Northeast Baptist," he said. "I have to do it. We have to get her over here. She's going to die if I don't do it."

Cindy agreed and found a bed at University of Texas Health Science Center of San Antonio. That was Thursday, September 2. We didn't even wait for an ambulance. My parents loaded me up in the car and drove me across San Antonio to University Hospital. It might have been the last time I would ride in a car. I, along with my parents, walked into the Surgical ICU, and I hopped up into my bed. Wordlessly, the staff watched, like we were a parade coming through, and then glanced at each other.

University Hospital was built in 1915. In 1968, its first class was admitted at the medical school. The campus is 100 acres, which is not enough land to hold the lives changed by the University of Texas Health Science

Center at San Antonio.

"Most of my patients don't *walk* in here," began Jennifer West, the nurse in charge.

That night, I called everyone whose number was saved in my cell phone. I left voicemails for several of my friends, which basically consisted of, "Hi! I'm having *brain surgery tomorrow*!"

By the way, cell phones are a big no-no in the hospital. Evidently they cause all the machines and monitors to wig out, and sometimes the sprinkler system goes off. I called Carrie and Tanya, my two best friends in North Dakota and Minnesota, and I left voicemail for my pal Jeff.

"Hi Jeffy, it's me. I'm having brain surgery tomorrow. Have a great weekend!"

He informed me later to *never* leave him a voicemail like that again. If he didn't want the voicemail, he should answer the phone. Some people enjoy my voicemails. I sing a lot.

Chaplains Harris and Taylor were there, praying with us. The phone in my room rang and Chaplain Taylor answered it. It was Tom, from the radio station.

"Why is the chaplain answering the phone?" Tom

demanded. He thought I'd already passed.

"Can I come see you?" I told him yes, but he'd better hurry, because I was about to have my haircut. I told him I would donate it to him, my intentionally bald friend.

Soon, Dr. Bogaev came in to meet my parents and me.

"Sunny Dee," Dr. Bogaev said, "That's you?" I nodded. "Which side is numb?" I told him it was my left side, and wondered if someone hadn't already told him that, but appreciated that he was double-checking, since he was about to go inside my head.

"In the morning, we're going to start the incision here at the top of your forehead, and come around like a backwards question mark," Dr. Bogaev began. Pausing, and raising an eyebrow at me from the foot of my bed, he asked, "Do you want to hear this?"

Mom looked at me, gauging my level of sedation and her own level of comfort.

"I don't think Deanna and I want to hear this right now," she said. "After it's all over, I want to hear every detail. But not now. If you'd like to take Curt into the hall and explain to him, that would be good," Mom said.

Dad nodded and indicated he was very interested in the craniotomy and resection plans. He and Dr. Bogaev grabbed my stack of MRI scans and disappeared to a room somewhere in the hospital with a light wall, where they could discuss the tumor at length.

In that quiet moment, my mom bent down to me, face to face.

"Are you scared?" she asked.

"No. Are you scared?"

"No," she said.

And we really weren't. I didn't feel worried or scared. I think when a person is so very near death or danger, and we give it all to Him, God grants us a peace, in order to make whatever's going to happen easier. Time slows down for us when we put ourselves in God's hands.

Hey, I had a brain tumor. There was a reason for all that madness. I had gone from being completely together and totally in control a few years prior to being so sick and so nervous all the time. I'm still relieved there was a reason for all that. I'm relieved every day.

My co-worker Tom brought me a chocolate chip

Frappuccino and a dense espresso brownie. Thinking it might be my last meal, he sweet-talked the nurses in the hallway,

"Please, it's all she wants." He takes every opportunity to sweet-talk nurses, waitresses, and flight attendants.

Most patients in the Surgical ICU don't get to have Starbucks coffee.

"Why are y'all bein' so nice?" I grinned. "Do I have a brain tumor or something?"

"Hey, can I pick your brain?" my mom kept joking. "Just the bad stuff."

"Are we shaving my head yet?" I kept asking of no one in particular. *Come on; let's get to the fun part.* I was still on some pretty hefty steroids for the pain, and eventually a Dr. Nitin came into the room. All I saw of him was his nametag, with my head against his chest as he worked on my hair.

Dr. Nitin asked if I wanted all of my head shaved, or just the side on which they would be operating. I told him to go ahead and take it all. I'm not living the lifestyle of lopsided haircuts. I do an 80s show, but I don't have to dress the part of Flock of Seagulls. From somewhere behind me, I heard my dad say, Yeah.

THAT'S my girl."

My dad is the type of guy who plays it pretty close to the vest. He had never said that before in my life. I will live on that sentence forever. Dads need to know their encouragement matters.

Dr. Nitin proceeded to take off two feet of thick, freshly permed (eighty bucks two weeks before!) "cheerleader hair.

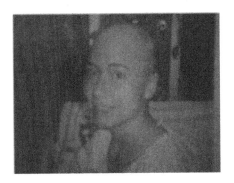

"They gave the hair to my mom in two "Biohazard" bags, because she wanted to use it in making a doll with

a lot of hair. She calls them "Gettin' Good Dolls," which look like children facing the wall and covering their faces. I imagine there were several times over the previous couple of years that she'd have loved to sit me in a corner until I "got good."

My housemate Brent was there for the haircut. He said Sinead O'Connor didn't have "nothin'" on me, bald with big eyes.

Then Dr. Nitin glued several plastic things onto my cranium (they resembled those hard plastic eyes on stuffed toys), which, after an MRI, would aid in creating a map for Dr. Bogaev to use in planning my surgery. This technology was less than a year old! I thought I looked like Darth Maul, from Star Wars!

My mom told me to make a list of all the email addresses I could remember. She went to Bakers' that night and sent out an email calling for prayer, and to let everyone know what was going on. After that email explained my voicemail messages, I'm sure a lot of those friends understood why I had been going off the deep end when they heard about the tumor. That makes me feel a little better about my last year of college.

I woke up alone in the hospital. Mom and Dad were at Grammy and Grampy Baker's. The energy of the last two days was replaced by the quiet buzzing of monitors and nurses' feet shuffling up and down the hallway.

I kept feeling my head. It felt like a little boy's haircut, with all of my hair clipped off like a new puppy. It reminded me of a little boy I babysat back when I was in high school. Ryan would run over to me in church on Sunday mornings before service began, and lean his head over, to have me feel the top of his head whenever he had a fresh haircut. Right away this September morning, I don't think I grasped that this was *my* haircut.

A stout German nurse named Bridget came in and took my vital statistics. She told me to remove my "underwears," and then there would be a lot of waiting for an Operating Room suite to become available. Mom and Dad arrived.

Then Pisamin came to get me. Pisamin was the nurse who wheeled me to the OR. Her name sounds like PIECE OF MIND. She was pleasant and brought calm to the room.

I remember being on a gurney, and my parents got to walk alongside me. When we got downstairs in the hospital, the clock on the wall read 10:20. Pisamin said this spot was the "Goodbye Place. This is the Hugs and Kisses Place." I got goodbye hugs and kisses from Mom and Dad. Then they wheeled me in.

I was thinking about my friend Jim taking me on a rollercoaster for the first time. The ride began. *Oh no, I've changed my mind, I ever-so gently tried to sit up. I don't want to get on. I guess it's too late now. The cart is in motion.*

Something happened. I remember a scrub-wearing guy putting the black mask over my mouth and nose to begin the anesthesia. Before the mask went on, I jokingly asked him if I should count backward from one hundred, like they make you do when you get your wisdom teeth out. I had my wisdom teeth out two Christmases before, in the hopes that it would help with the horrendous headaches I'd been having.

"If you want," he shrugged, not looking at me as he answered. I took a deep breath, and I made it to 98.

I saw colors, like a rainbow, only not a rainbow. It was welcoming and warm and something like a bright misty stained glass window with the sun shining through on Sunday morning, or sort of a kaleidoscope. There was a lot of yellow, green and blue. A little red. I walked through it. I couldn't not.

Then I felt like someone was holding me very tightly, so I couldn't breathe.
There were people everywhere. It was like Grand Central Station, but all in white. The light was everywhere. Then the urgency of it all paused, like it was on videotape or something. I rounded a dark corner, feeling a stone wall on my left hand, and a coolness crossed my face, like walking to school on a

frosty, foggy morning in the autumn in North Dakota. It got really quiet, and was all white and quiet, but it wasn't really like a room. It really felt like I was in my front yard, in Washburn, North Dakota, on a brisk fall morning. There was some fog coming up from the ground. I saw a man in knee-length jean shorts and an olive green t-shirt, wearing socks with his sandals. At the time I thought it was my dad, but he looked years younger. His mustache and hair were a little longer. I don't think anyone dresses like that for surgery. Did Dr. Bogaev have my dad scrub in for my operation? I could believe that.

I let go of the cold rock wall I was holding onto and stepped down off the cool stone path I was on, and was surprised to feel a crunchy grass met my feet. Okay, wait, that made sense. If the air was that cool when it hit on my cheeks, the grass would be crunchy. The grass felt exactly like the dew had frozen overnight, as it does in the autumn, when winter warns us of his impending stay. I looked up at Dad. His jaw clenched, and the movement on the side of his head made his glasses shift ever-so slightly. I knew this was not my assignment right now. I was supposed to be doing something else. Dishes, maybe. I backed up onto the stone path.

There is someone who greets you in Heaven, and everyone else rushes around in a happy way, because they are excited. They say hello, and hug you, make no mistake. The greeter among the Heavenly host-- I don't know who that was, but he sure looked a lot like Dad.

Mom is convinced I have about ten thousand guardian angels, and they have to work in shifts, because I keep wearing them out.

One friend suggested to me that man must have been Jesus. It is said we assign traits to our Heavenly Father based on how we feel about, fear, or relate to our Earthly Father.

I promise you, He is there. It is beautiful. It feels amazing. They are waiting to greet us.

On a summer Sunday evening, nearly a year later, at Dr. B's house for a dinner of surf and turf, he told me the story of losing my vitals just after administering the anesthetic, because of the swelling of the tumor around my brain stem.

'Pre-death conditions," Dr. Bogaev confirmed, while grilling sea bass at his home.

Scientific studies recently supported the near-death experience, or NDE. Science still doesn't know what to make of my airy stained-glass entry, or the stone hallway, or even the gathering of white-clad greeters in the fresh air that met me that day. I will tell you, it is the easiest moment I ever had, and I don't know how long I was there. It was probably only a moment. I had surgery on a Saturday. I fully awoke on a Tuesday. I am the most blessed person we know.

My friend Michael recently received a new kidney, and while talking with him about his surgery and different aspects of his hospitalization, we got around to his NDE. I told him the Doorway is a Stained Glass Window. He said, "I know!"

CHAPTER SIX

John 15:13 "Greater love hath no man than this, that a man lay down his life for his friends."

The next thing I knew, I heard Tanya talking to me. Tanya was my college roommate. I was listening to her tell me about having an ultrasound. She was six months pregnant and she was saying that she got really big, really fast, and if there were two babies in her tummy, I'd have to do double duty and be mommy to one while being auntie to the other.

"No, no," I said, patting her stomach. I was thinking, *okay, this is a dream. There is no way Tanya is in Texas. Furthermore, I am too tired to babysit.*

Next to Tanya, by my knees, I heard Carrie telling me,

"Hush. Don't talk." She has never been successful at shutting me up, and she's tried. Poor thing, I'm the talker of the gang, and Carrie has to put up with it when I want to jabber, because she is the voice of reason. But at that moment, I rolled my head over and went back to sleep.

In cartoons, when a character is bonked on the head with a big black anvil or a grand piano, they see stars and chirping birds swirling around. That is exactly how it is to wake up after sixteen hours of brain surgery and three days.

I remember hearing familiar voices, and trying to open my eyes. I saw just about everyone I knew in Texas: people from work, my housemate Brent, two English ladies from my church talking about scones and tea. I saw my co-workers Naomi and Norma waving from the foot of the bed, and a great big stuffed Winnie the Pooh. Darleen, a fellow radio personality, was right up close to the head of my bed. She'd come up near my shoulder, so I didn't have to focus too hard, and she'd brought me a stuffed lion. Grammy Baker put a silver angel bracelet on my right wrist and kissed the back of my hand.

Those ICU people only want two visitors in any patient room at a time. They didn't know *my* people until then, but when they saw the long-haired rockers from the station rolling in, they just waved them toward my room. They'd given up on rules.

I was very cranky with my adoring mother, who was trying to tickle me awake. Did she not *know* that I had one foot and my nose in Heaven? She was just trying to wake me up, so the alarms would quit going off. My intracranial pressure was too high. I like to set off bells and whistles. Ask anybody.

At one point early on, I heard the doctor talking to my parents about a post-op CT scan. I couldn't move or talk, but I panicked. I did not want to go inside the magnet just then.

"CT scan, please," I whispered. "Not an MRI."

"Yes," he assured me. "We're going to do a CT scan."

I was so cold in Radiology, and someone put a warm blanket over me. You know the one. The blanket out of the special blanket warmer you wish you had in your house. It felt awesome. I presumed it was a redheaded male nurse or an MRI technician who helped me with this, and I hoarsely whispered, "Thank you for helping me."

The person with the blanket was my own world-renowned neurosurgeon, Dr. Bogaev. The nurses cried.

Then Mom was saying my name.

"Virgil and Tom are here. Can you wake up?"

I thought, "Wow! They sent management in! It must almost be my funeral or something! I am so tired, but... Oh, shoot, am I *on the air???*"

Try to get normal, I thought. Try to wake up and get normal. I do recall Virgil's wonderfully booming voice. I couldn't open my eyes to visit.

In the next few days, during my waking moments, I slowly became more aware of what was going on.

"Humph, I guess that really all happened," I thought. I wasn't aware of the extent of my situation, but I knew I had a lot of work ahead of me, and I had an urge to talk to my grandpa.

There were lots of flowers and everything was really animated. When you are down and very nearly out, the family of your heart will bribe nurses with chocolate. You will be taken care of.

All these people were coming to watch me sleep. Hope didn't snore. Oh baby, I am *not* a cute girl on steroids and with a swollen, purple, bald head. *Not* a cute girl.

There is a lot of photographic evidence of that.

And then Mom told me Carrie and Tanya had really been there. I was so sad that they came all that way and I didn't even get to talk with them, because it was so hard to live across the country from my best friends.

"You talked to me," Carrie said when she called the hospital one night. "I kept telling you not to try to talk."

That sounded familiar.

"Jennifer has a cowboy name," I told my mom over and over, laughing, referring to Nurse Jennifer West. Jennifer was my immediate post-op caretaker. She decorated a scrubs cap with hearts and smiley faces, to cover some of the incision. She fed me and bathed me, and listened patiently while I tried to speak. When my parents would arrive for visiting hours, and Mom would ask if I had eaten breakfast, my answer would save me from saying extraneous words.

"Jennifer knows."

"Jennifer has a cowboy name." I'll bet at that point they thought I was not going to be mentally twenty-three years old again. I still think it's funny. I can call her on the phone and ask, "Hi, is this *Jennifer With the Cowboy Name?"* And she knows it's me. She didn't wear me out by making me take those first few weeks.

I couldn't use my tongue to pronounce "country singer," so merely pronouncing lip words like "cowboy name" would have to do.

Most of my friends, recently out of college and struggling to get established in the world, cannot afford an impromptu vacation.

The fact that Carrie and Tanya thought nothing of coming to San Antonio right away just blows my mind. A week later, two more college friends, Heather and Amanda, flew in. They showered me with gifts. I had stuffed toys, big NDSU latte mugs, an NDSU hat, bath products and even a radio, because they knew I'd need to listen. I know that their immediate trip here probably set them back in their financial planning. I pray I am as good and selfless a friend.

So there I was in the hospital, and every time some poor, unsuspecting doctor came around to do rounds, I'd ask them how brain tumors grew... well, they didn't know. Less than two cents of every dollar given for cancer research goes toward brain cancer. This swollen, purple, 23-yr-old bald thing was whispering these questions, like, "How did it start?"

Finally, one doctor got close enough to my head to hear

me whispering.

The poor man had walked in and amusedly muttered, "Well. Welcome to the Hundred Acre Wood," for my cohorts had FILLED the place with Winnie-the-Pooh and Friends.

"We don't know," he said. "Something got in there and it just began."

"Like an oyster grows a pearl?" I whispered.

At the time, in my mind, I thought I was speaking. I was whispering. Very, very quietly and in monotone. I had no lung capacity to speak of, and I am sure it took a lot of patience to gather THAT sentence from me.

"Say it again," he said, very close to my face so he could hear me. "One more time."

When he caught the gist of what I was trying to communicate, he smiled.

"Yes. Like a pearl."

So, the tape was looping around in my head that my brain tumor was like some pearl, and had started from a figurative grain of sand. And that is how I explained it to myself. Being in the hospital was bad at night. After visiting hours, when Mom and everyone would leave, the nurses turned out the lights. In the darkness, it felt like being buried alive. My left side was unable to move. I never want to do that again. I still sleep with lights on.

Ann, one of my favorite ICU nurses, said to me one evening,

"It's okay to cry. It's called 'Sundowner Syndrome.' Everyone gets sad in the hospital at night.'"

But I didn't cry. I didn't think enough to cry then. I was beyond crying. I couldn't cry anyway. I could not make tears form in my eyes. I didn't have the lung capacity to breathe fully, and I could not speak above a monotone whisper. I wasn't going to waste air by sobbing.

When Dr. Bogaev would come by my room on his rounds, he asked me to frown for him. Then he would ask me to smile, really big. "Let's see your teeth," he said. You mean, the teeth I haven't brushed in a week? SMILE! AAAAHHH! This was so he could see if my facial muscles were all connected correctly, after he had peeled off half of my face and put it back. I could only smile with the right side of my face, but I became good at frowning, in jest.

"Wow, look at that! That's fine, real fi-ine." He'd say in his Arkansas accent, making a big deal out of my facial muscles. If he was happy, that meant all the muscles were reattached correctly and maybe I didn't look as scary as I felt. I was happy, too.

My mom had been telling me about a nineteen-year-old girl in the next room who was completely broken. She had been in an auto accident and had broken arms, legs, collarbones and a shattered pelvis. Her name is Genny.

"Does Genny cry when her mother leaves?" I managed to whisper to Laura, one of the nurses who came in at night. I begged Laura for my car keys and my phone. I begged Laura to let me get up. I hadn't even tried getting up at that point, so I don't know how I would have felt about it when I realized I couldn't.

"No," she said crisply, as she walked out of the room. "Genny doesn't cry."

I felt horrible that I was obviously annoying her, and I

would apologize profusely.

"I'm sorry. I'm so sorry. I'm just so tired tonight. I'm sorry."

I was whisper-talking the apology as loudly as possible, since Laura had already left my room, but due to the fact that I had weak lung capacity, and she was probably very busy anyway, no one could hear me. I could not move.

My arms were restrained to either side of my hospital bed, and when I came to that realization, it began to bother me very much, because I started to feel like I was drowning. Maybe I was buried. The room was very dark.

I had nightmares. Vampires surrounded me, and I thought I was at some kind of twisted blood drive. I felt weak and was calling for my brother Travis. See, my calling out was barely a whisper, and Travis wouldn't answer me. It took every bit of my lung capacity to say…one…word…at…a…time. I was convinced that I was being held captive by vampires in Grand Forks, North Dakota, and that Travis was there, somewhere, and I had to get him back to Fargo for his classes. I was in great distress that night, because I could not find my car keys, and I was supposed to be responsible for Travis.

I was being a terrible big sister, which would reflect poorly on his college career. In these visions, I thought I saw my friend Mike's white Grand Am parked directly outside of my window. I was so confused as to why Mike wasn't bounding in the door to rescue me. I felt completely abandoned.

I think that vampire dream had to do with nurses taking a lot of blood, often, and the darkness in which I lived.

One eye was swollen shut, and the other side of my face was numb and tingly. Meanwhile, my arms were strapped to both sides of the bed. All we could do was give it time.

I thought I was in some kind of community hospital ward, with other patients, lying next to each other. I couldn't roll myself over to see who was lying beside me. Whomever it was, I was reasonably sure they weren't there in the daytime, when everyone else was.

Looking at pictures, I see it was one of the big stuffed Pooh bears that somebody brought me! Boy, and for so long I've thought, *How campy, that they just flop bodies here and there. What kind of place is this? Where have they left me?*

That's funny! Someone snuggled a Pooh bea
me and I've been afraid of it all this time. My
was too weak to see peripherally, and my rig
not really seeing anything, due to the third ne
from the operation. It was dark. Dark.

CHAPTER SEVEN

PT stands for Pretty Tolerable

The physical therapists began to come around to try to
get me moving. I really didn't like that first pair of
physical therapists, The Nickel Brothers. This is
significant, because this first PT session was nearing
NDSU Homecoming, and I first thought of The Nickel
Trophy. I hoped they'd be wonderful, that I would
really like them, and I could have a great Nickel Story.
No.

I thought they were mean, treating me as though I were
being a noncompliant, lazy patient. They lectured me
on attitude, while I struggled to keep my eyes open. I

decided not to waste any precious breath explaining to these two guys that they didn't know me, *my* attitude, and it wasn't that I just *wouldn't* do it. I absolutely *could not* move my left arm or leg. Yet. Seriously, was I their first patient ever?

"You really work at a radio station?" One of the evil physical therapy twins asked, condescendingly. "You push buttons and stuff?"

Yeah, I push buttons. In real life, I talk, too. A lot.

Dr. Bogaev told me the difference in hemiplegia and hemiparesis, is that with one, you're very weak on one side. Hemiparesis means paralyzed. I told them my arm was being "fat and lazy," because steroids puff you up a lot. If only I could breathe. The PT gargoyles did not return after the second session, with their insulting commentary on whom I was obviously not.

I tried to move, but nothing would respond. There would be a new plan. I thought really hard about it all the time. At night, when it was dark, I thought so hard about moving, that sometimes I thought I actually was able to. I imagined I was doing a scissors kick, like in swimming lessons when I was ten years old. I was the best one in the class.

"Now everybody watch Deanna," the lifeguards would

say, using my first name, and having me swim the American crawl or the scissors kick the length of the pool in our little town. "That's how you do it."

I can still feel the coolness of the sheets. *Why couldn't I move during the day, and show Dr. Bogaev?*

My mom would keep friends and family updated almost daily on email. In those days, there was no social media. We had hotmail and yahoo. Google hadn't even become a Thing.

Mom would print out their emails and bring them to the hospital and read them to me. I loved that. I *so* looked forward to it. Keeping in touch with my friends is so vital to me. Mom was keeping me connected. She read me cards and letters. She quizzed me on the names of the flowers in the floral arrangements.

Sunflower, sunflower, rose, daisy, bird of paradise.

Two weeks after surgery, I was moved to a rehabilitation hospital down Medical Drive from University Hospital in San Antonio. It's called Warm Springs. I envisioned hot tubs and hoped for gorgeous male nurses in togas, feeding me grapes. No such luck. It sounds very inviting, unless you *have* to be there. If you are paralyzed on one side of your body, and the other side is strapped to the bed, and you can't move, drink, pee, or talk on the phone by yourself, then you don't want to be anywhere.

 My first night, I lay awake looking at the glow of streetlights out my window and San Antonio beyond. Thank Heaven they put me by the window! I didn't sleep a wink. I couldn't move to get comfortable, my back hurt and I kept thinking,

"If I bother Mom enough tomorrow, she'll take me home with her."

Every few hours, a group of nurses would come in to turn me over. I'm sure they were on a schedule, and had other patients to turn, but they didn't ask me if they had me in an okay position. I recall feeling very embarrassed and sort of inwardly upset that I was being turned over like a fish, to prevent bedsores. I knew what they were doing. I knew why they were doing it. But I tried to be compliant and not complain. I did not want to risk a negative notation in my chart. I wanted to get on their good side.

 Sometimes I would pretend to be sleeping when they came around. I couldn't say much to them at that juncture, anyway. They just turned me over, whether it was comfortable or not, and sometimes my face met my pillow in a precarious way. I couldn't move at all to get into a better spot; hence, the stiff, aching back and difficulty breathing. I'd never been so afraid. My back was twisted and my face was in the pillow. I was suffocating.

"You okay, baby?" My roommate, Nona, hit her nurse call button, because she knew I wasn't. Nona is an older black woman with more motherly instinct than most humans. A nurse, Lisa, rushed in.

"She can't breathe or something," Nona told Lisa, who immediately got me situated, and life became better from that moment on.

I wish I could have spoken more, because I would have loved to talk to Ms. Nona. At the risk of making the rehab hospital sound like a prison, Ms. Nona was in for back surgery. She was doing time for spinal stenosis. Thank God we were put together in Room 415. I appreciate the guardian angel.

They had a lot of agency nurses, who would work one day a week, and were unfamiliar with the patients.

One nurse reached for my left arm and Mom screamed, "Don't pull on her left arm, you'll pull it out of the shoulder socket!"

Hence, to this day, my left bra strap falls off my shoulder. Not a huge deal, I suppose. I just need to work on my posture more than most.

In the morning, a nurse came to get me up and to the "feeding group." That was an unforgettable experience. First of all, up until that point, I hadn't gotten up. I thought, *That's a new one. I don't do that. I don't get out of bed. I'd like to, but I just don't think it's possible.*

It was quite a dizzying transition, from lying down to sitting up. They put me in a wheelchair, which I was kind of excited about, because it denoted mobility. I was dressed, and wheeled down the hallway to a room with several round tables. I did not see anyone my own age. There were several elderly people there, and I began to feel like I had been put in a nursing home. *Oh no, where have they left me?*

Then, when I didn't eat much of my breakfast, and asked to be excused, a nurse who was writing down the percentage of my meal I *had* eaten told me, in thee most Southern accent you've ever heard, I was breaking her little heart by not eating any more of that good food. My lung capacity and verbal skills still had a long way to go, so I just told her I wasn't hungry, and looked downward. I didn't want to try to discuss too much more about it.

In fact, the problem was, *I couldn't feed myself.* It was embarrassing and I didn't have the energy to fight, especially if there were people around. My right eye was lazy from the operation, giving me double vision. My horrible depth perception made it nearly impossible to navigate a spoon or cup to my mouth. Besides, there was some kind of bland hot cereal on my tray, and I could not tear open a sugar packet to sweeten it, because I couldn't use both hands. I could not whisper loudly and clearly enough to ask for help with the sugar. I wanted to sink into the floor. Please stop trying to talk me into another attempt at eating. *I'm not hungry.* In my head, I was thinking, "because it's too hard."

When the dining attendants understand you're not going to eat, they wheel you up to the hallway. Then, there was a lot of waiting. They would place the patients up along the hallway into a long line opposite the nurses' station. When someone had time, they would wheel us back to our rooms, one at a time.

I couldn't go alone. With only one arm and one leg, I would only go in circles, not to mention the impossible incline of the hallway back to Room 415. Later on in my stay, I would get brave, and try to wheel myself. It meant crashing into the wall at the nurses' station, with my one hand and one leg, and being put back in line. Sometimes, at the end of the line.

So we all waited. And waited. I tried reading the clock so I would know how long it was taking, but I could not comprehend the numbers yet. The clock looked like the numbers were swirly and jumbled. Looking at the clock for long made me feel sick.

Charolette, Cognitive and Speech Therapy, would work on that with me. Often, my wheelchair was put next to this young man in a very high wheelchair, with one leg sticking out in front. His name was Joe, and he was in pretty bad shape. He moaned and yelled a lot, sometimes all night long. His cries echoed down the hall. One morning, as harshly as my lungs would allow, I whispered at Joe.

"Shhhh! What gives *you* the right to yell? Nobody's happy. Just hush!"

Later, I learned why Joe cried all the time. He was only nineteen, and was riding his bike one day, months before. At a stop sign, he was run over by a volunteer fireman. The man was in a pickup truck on his way to a fire.

Joe had a feeding tube in his stomach, and only got to eat breakfast by his mouth. The rest of the time, he was fed shakes through the tube. So he was hungry. Joe was a typical, hungry teenager beneath his injuries. That's why poor Joe cried.

I was so sorry. I felt horrible for having admonished Joe. We take so much for granted, and simply the fact that I could chew and swallow food felt like a miracle to me.

I did everything I could to get out of the hospital. Cards and letters continued to pour in, and I found the knowledge that people were praying for me very inspirational.

The faith of my loved ones, people who sincerely cared about me, made me well. I had no idea all those people cared about me. I heard and read things most people only say at funerals. *That's* why I walk again. If they all really believed in me that much, I could do anything.

If I get sad or lonely, or just think I can't do it anymore, I reread my get well cards.

Mark 11:52 "And Jesus said, 'Go your way; your faith has made you well.'"

The first sentence I could say very well was, "I'm amazing." And why not? Everyone told me I was – my physical therapists, the nurses, my doting mother, my radio people, and the therapists. Those words didn't require a lot of tongue movement. My tongue was still not moving, anyway. You only need your lips to pronounce yourself amazing. My lips were fine.

Say something often enough, and you will be able to get through physical therapy, maybe even occupational therapy. Perhaps, if you believe in your amazingness, you will be able to navigate a fork or a coffee cup to your mouth, and thereby feed yourself. Amazing covers a lot of ground, once it wells up inside of you.

Remember that ex-boyfriend from college? The one who'd told me I was no fun when my body went numb and my heart was palpitating, and I thought I was going to die? He heard through the radio grapevine that I was in the hospital, and called one night while the nurses were getting me set up to watch the FRIENDS premiere. Even one of the other patients came to my room to watch with me, Nona and Mom. Our room was definitely the social hub of Warm Springs Rehabilitation Hospital.Her name was Jennifer.

So ex-boyfriend man. I suppose he had called the radio station and my good friend Larry Chase, who was keeping the good times rolling on my 80s show, sang like a bird about where I was. Ex-Boyfriend Man tracked me down, even to this hospital, even to Room 415B.

He said, "Gee, it sounds like you've been to the dentist. What, did they take away your alphabet brain cell?"

He laughed. He was trying to be funny. Being supremely disgusted with this joke, and unwilling to let this opportunity pass by, I let a moment of silent lucidity sink in, while I mustered up everything I had to deliver my indignant response.

In some kind of slurring way, I told him, "If I'd hung around you any longer I wouldn't have *any* brain cells left."

"Hey, that's pretty good," he laughed. I think I said goodbye before I hung up. Maybe I just hung up. Eyerolling was too painful at that stage of the game.

I was so hurt and self-conscious after that. It probably wasn't the most compassionate move to ring someone up following brain surgery and boil it down to a shot of Novocain. Therapy took such a very long time with my left hand. In the morning, an attendant asked me if I wanted sugar in my tea, and I said, "Yes. Two please, to keep me sweet-tempered."

She asked me, "HUH? What are you saying?" I repeated, "Two, please, to keep me sweet-tempered." She turned around and hollered to the other attendants in the feeding group, who were all helping other patients with their breakfasts. "I can't understand her. What's she trying to say?"

I was so embarrassed. *Oh my goodness, I am a communicator, and this woman can't understand me. What am I going to do? I make a living by talking.*

Charolette, my Speech and Cognitive Therapist, knew what she was doing when she had sessions with me. I think she had it on her heart that every moment I spent with her was another chance to regain a fraction of my life, my career, my former self. Physical Therapists give extra attention to injured athletes. I would not only need my speech therapy to regain regular speech, but I was a Radio Personality, in a huge city, with a fun show. I needed Charolette to help me if I ever hoped to get back to that. I had been a speech champion in high school and college. Charolette and I read books, did complex math problems, and we talked. A lot.

A week or two later, Ex-Boyfriend Man called again.

He asked, "How are you?"

"I'm amazing."

"Boy, you sound really good."

"I'm amazing."

"No, I mean, *really* good."

"I'm amazing." I glanced up, as my dear friend

Angelita from the radio station entered the room for FRIENDS Night. "And I have to go."

Hanging up that phone was perhaps the most strengthening exercise I could have done for myself in that relationship.

Mark 5:41 - "Taking her by the hand, he said to her, 'Little girl, I say to you, arise.'"

Grammy and Grampy Baker are a dear couple at my church in San Antonio. They came right away to my bedside and Grammy wrapped a silver angel bracelet around my right wrist and kissed the back of my hand. It was beautiful.

My arms were so bruised from the IVs, and we noticed what we thought to be a strange phenomenon. Along the line where my silver angel bracelet fell, my skin had healed. The bruising had completely gone away. On their next visit, I asked Grammy to move the angel over to my unmoving left arm, because that one needed healing too. I had become more aware of my situation and condition, according to my chart notes and Dr. Leonard, the physical therapy doctor.

One morning, about two weeks into my stay at Warm Springs Rehabilitation Hospital, while waiting for someone to wheel me from the feeding group area back to my room, I felt an involuntary muscle spasm cause my leg to jump. It gave me so much hope. I stared at my leg, willing it to jump again. I think I cried out, and a nurse came running. The therapists jumped on this opportunity, if nerves were firing, and I henceforth had a full therapy schedule.

"I just knew it would move," I thought. "Give me a few more weeks, I'll be as good as new."

That was the Sunday morning Chaplain Harris came in after church to tell me there had been a prayer meeting the night before, and the building was on fire praying for my left arm and left leg.

"Well, then I should show you what I can do today." I raised my left arm and left leg about two inches off my bed. To me, it felt like I was punching and kicking the sky. He almost fainted, then jumped up and ran around the room hollering "Praise Jesus! Thank you, Lord!"

I suppose I could talk about how much I really did not like being incapacitated in a rehabilitation hospital. Eva, the medication nurse was plain *scary*, and sometimes the physical therapy was grueling. But I can't dwell on that side of it too much, because I adore the therapists I had there.

I loved when my physical therapist, Nori, would have

me try to walk ten feet along a set of parallel bars, holding onto me as I held onto the bars with each step. The parallel bars meant standing. Standing meant walking. Walking meant recovery. Recovery meant going home. My mom teased Nori about looking like Jennifer Beal from "Flashdance." I could hear the theme music from *Rocky* in my head. Yeah, *bring it on.*

The therapists would all ask me, "Do you want to rest? Do you want some water? Do you want to do more?"

"More," I managed to say. *Let me just do more until I'm strong enough to go home.*

That, I have on video. It isn't easy to watch.

Occupational therapy, for my left arm, and my left hand, was a bit tougher, because it involved finer motor skills. I would try so hard to slide my arm in an arc on a table in front of me, but sometimes it honestly hurt my head, I was thinking so hard. I did not understand the disconnect between my brain and the left side of my body. Why was nothing over there moving? Lorenzo and Adriana would have made me stop if I said it hurt. I did almost cry *just once*, but I didn't want to show any weakness.

I'm tougher than you think. Let me do more until I can

go home.

When my hand-to-mouth skills got a little better, Charolette, my speech and cognitive therapist, brought me a brownie one day and observed while I took a bite and swallowed it successfully. I thought I was just getting an extra dessert, like I deserved a treat for working so hard.

"Ok, you can have your meals in your room. I'll write the order."

God bless her. Charolette the Angel saved me from the feeding group! I was making progress.

"You know if you'd had problems swallowing, I wouldn't have," she says, these days.

Yeah, yeah, I think to myself, but you did.

Somebody from the radio station came to visit everyday. Brian Kendall worked the night show at the rock station down the hall. He's my work brother. Walks me to my car at midnight, and buys me dinner. Tries to get me to go out and listen to bands, but I'm a goody two shoes and I wear Winnie-the-Pooh clothes, so I'm not going out after midnight. I'm going home to watch Conan O'Brien. Brian looks like a rock and roll star, and seems a little surprising visiting a hospital religiously. But he was always there, smile sparkling and eyes dancing. He brought me pizza, because he knows what I like.

One day, we had pizza and Mom took a piece down the hall to Joe.

"Pizza," he was able to say. "More."

That was a breakthrough for Joe. This nineteen-year-old kid couldn't talk, and everyone accepted that. But he knew, "pizza."

That made him so happy. He really liked my mom after that. It was like a miracle, to finally see some response out of him. And all it took was some pizza.

One evening, Mom and Dad were still in my room visiting Nona and me. I'm kind of a night person, and a morning person. Blame it on the radio. Something in my head insisted that I tell her, "Pollo Jack."

Mom made me repeat those words a dozen times, because I was still not speaking very well. It must have sounded something like I was breathing out, "pojack." She apologized, but she just did not know what that meant.

She got really close to my face, because she couldn't

hear my monotone whispering. "Honey, I don't know what you're saying."

"Ask BK." I knew that my radio brother could clear this up in an instant.

"I don't have BK's number."

So I gave it to her. BK would be on the air now, and my eyes could not yet read the numbers on a clock, but I could rattle off the super-secret KISS hotline phone number.

Mom dialed the digits, and sure enough, Brian Kendall answered.

"She keeps saying, 'Pollo Jack.' What does that mean?" my mother asked my rock-and-roll work brother. Brian Kendall laughed, giggled and chortled. Mom held the phone so I could hear. "It means she's hungry! She wants the Pollo Jack Enchilada Dinner from Taco Cabana!"

BK knows how to order food. As the 7 to midnight radio personalities on sister stations, we ate dinner together most evenings, and he heard me sing that commercial for two months before I went into the hospital. Chicken Cheese Enchiladas were one of the first things I requested, then later in the week he showed up with that pizza. A girl must get awfully hungry, being unable to feed herself.

On another day, Radio Engineer Robert brought my parents a gift certificate to a local steakhouse. My parents went on a date, and I asked them to please bring me some Range Rattlers.

"Some WHAT?!" My poor mother. She very often does not know what I'm talking about. Numero Uno: I was difficult to understand. Dos: Was this a real menu item, or did I make up these things in my head? I am pretty creative, after all. When they returned from dinner to help get me ready for bed that night, my momma had not let me down. She indeed had a Styrofoam from the restaurant with Range Rattlers, and I was able to feed myself. We're talking seafood salad, inside a jalapeno, with the shrimp tail, breaded and deep-friend. Glorious. Not for the delicate palate. Most certainly for me. I like my coffee, food, and boys to be hot.

There were lots of flowers and everything was really animated. Ric and the production department from the radio station brought a whole chocolate cake. On the cake was written, "Get well, Josie *y los Gatos* (and the cats)." The nurses enjoyed the cake immensely. When you are down and very nearly out, the family of your heart will bribe nurses with chocolate. You will be taken care of.   All these people were coming to watch me sleep. Hope I didn't snore. I am *not* a cute girl on steroids and with a swollen, purple eye.

After five weeks, with the help of a cane, dressed in my Winnie-the-Pooh and Tigger clothes, I walked slowly out the front doors of that hospital. A bunch of my co-workers and my housemate Brent had come to celebrate the occasion. We released a bouquet of balloons into the bright blue Texas sky. They brought more flowers, and more stuffed animals. I was surrounded by love and support. I have that on video, too. It is wonderful to watch. News of my release (and the balloon release) was simultaneously shared on the local NBC magazine show, San Antonio Living, thanks to Sonny Melendrez.

We all went for Chinese immediately.

I went home with my parents to Copperas Cove for several weeks. I couldn't live alone just yet.

I had outpatient physical, occupational and speech therapy at Health South in Killeen, Texas. On my first day with the speech therapist, she did a routine evaluation in which she asked me to say a lot of things. Holding up her wristwatch, she asked me to name as many animals as I could in sixty seconds.

"Do you want them in alphabetical order?" I asked.

The look of horror that flashed across her face was worth my joke. "They didn't make you do it in alphabetical order at the hospital, did they?" she gasped.

No. I had seen that in the movie *Phenomenon*, and was in a crazy, showy mood. "Aardvark, bat, cat, dog, elephant, ferret, horse, giraffe..."

Then came time for the physical therapies.

"Can you do ten more?" asked Roslyn, my soldier physical therapist. She stopped herself when I nodded, and told me I needed a t-shirt that reads, "Yeah, I can do ten more!" I told her I worked in Radio, and I need another t-shirt like I need another hole in my head.

After two weeks, my speech therapist discharged me. She said she couldn't help me get any better than I was at that point. To a lifelong communicator, this was the progress I had been waiting to hear. I wanted to go back to work. Virgil and Tom called and asked if I was able and would like to come back to my show. Initially, my back-to-work projection had was one year. This was a mere three months post-op.

I moved back to Brent's house in San Antonio in December. Thankfully, the radio station put me back on the air. It was coming. My life was coming back to me. I was on the air less than three months after an extensive brain operation. I just didn't want to stop talking. I summoned all of my independence and put myself back together again.

I can put up a pretty good fight. It's too late to give up and die. There is no choice. You just have to drive on.

Besides, I love life too much not to be living it. I am so thankful and in wonder of it all on a daily basis. I can walk! I'm not being hauled around in a wheelchair. I get to drive my own car, which I love.

I get to go wherever I want, whenever I want. I can go to the gym alone, and a physical therapist is not dictating my every move. I can have gourmet coffee every single day.

CHAPTER EIGHT

There are people in your life who bring you only good things.

A year after my operation, I went to North Dakota to see my friends and family, to prove that, indeed, I was alive and recovering. My parents had moved back there, close to the grandmas.

Of course I have my sad days. Sometimes I feel like it's a mountainous task, this "Quest for One Hundred Percent," and I'd like to snap my fingers and be perfectly well again. But I don't let those sad days snowball into sad weeks. I firmly believe you can talk yourself happy, or talk yourself sad. I can't talk myself into being so depressed I'll never come up for air again. I just have to remember there's a Light at the End of the Tunnel.

Other people
Seem to always get their
Wishes granted.
The pennies they toss into
Fountains there and here
Must be shinier
Somehow,
Than mine.
So I shine my pennies
Very bright,
And hold each one up
To the Light.
Sometimes I toss in a dime or two.
Sometimes I make a wish for you.

I think my wish
Is coming.
Someday, somehow, some way.
I think God knows
How I faithfully throw
My pennies in everyday.
And when my wish
Finally gets here,
It'll be bigger,
And bright as a star,
And all those Single-Wish-Penny-People
Will wonder
What kind of wish-pennies
My wish-pennies are.

4/5/01

Everyone marvels at how well I'm doing, how
quickly I recovered. Those people don't know that
my left toes don't move. But I can snap my left
fingers. I know that one of my lessons is patience,
but I think God knew if He wanted to teach me how
to be patient, He'd have to do it in a hurry.

I also know that I didn't go through all that to be left
so far from the finish line. Every day I feel my
struggling to get from place to place gets a little
easier. There must be something really wonderful
out there for me, and I am so excited thinking about
t. I certainly haven't reached my happy ending yet,

but it's coming. An old Chinese legend says, "A faithful heart makes wishes come true." I have faith. I don't think a person can go through something like this and *not* have a strong faith.

I met Dr. Bogaev's parents. I thanked them for having him. I think of all the lives impacted by a person who studied hard and perfected his craft. There really is no excuse to slack off. You could be saving someone's life with your art.

I heard a wonderful story. When Mrs. Bogaev was pregnant, she didn't hear any boys' names to which she was really attached. She saw a Winnie-the-Pooh movie, and the next day went into labor. When she had a bouncing baby boy, she was reminded of how she liked the name Christopher, as in Christopher Robin. While hearing this story, I'm wearing a Winnie-the-Pooh shirt. I suppose it's coincidence that in the Hundred Acre Wood, when there are skullosauruses to fight, Christopher Robin prevails over them. And in the real world, when there are skull-based brain tumors to fight, Christopher Bogaev slays them, too. I don't believe in coincidences. I believe in miracles, and that the Universe is unfolding as it should.

Dr. Bogaev sent me to an epilepsy specialist, Dr. Szabo, who studied my brain waves and told me I probably won't have epilepsy from here on out, even though there is a large injury to my brain. He asked about the history, or "when this all began."

When I told him about the numbing panic attacks in college, he said they sounded like small seizures. That was scary. I had been functioning really well. I was driving. I was working at the newspaper and the station. I was drinking alcohol at radio station events. I could have been dead at any moment if one of those struck me at the wrong time. What I thought had been panic attacks, and myself acting psychotic and depressed, were seizures. Moreover, I could have hurt someone else. I am so blessed to have arrived on Dr. Bogaev's doorstep at the right moment. Thanks, God!

By the spring of 2001, I noticed my eyes were giving me some problems, but I chalked it up to being a night radio jock. I had gotten a new burst of energy, and developed a habit of going to the gym early in the morning when it opened, and then slept until the soap operas began. This schedule worked fine for me. I didn't have to be at work until five or so in the afternoon.

I would go sometimes, to see the therapists and the nurses and visit the patients no one was visiting and talk to them. When I was in the hospital, I really hated the down time, when no one was there and I just stared at the ceiling tiles. Down time was rare, because my mom did a great job of sitting at my bedside almost every waking moment, but the few times I was alone, I sure didn't like it.

CHAPTER NINE

The summer of 2001, the radio automation trend hit my station. I panicked, having worked every day since I was sixteen, and searched the radio job websites. I applied for an opening in Atlantic City, and when my show ended at midnight one Friday night, exactly three years to the day from my first 80s show, I moved to New Jersey to start my new midday gig Monday. I would be doing young country middays. To me, this was a great opportunity to live near the ocean and to get close to New York; Radio Market Number One. We were so close, in fact, that on Sunday mornings, the station shotgunned into New York. I guess you might say I can check that one off my bucket list.

I had a cute apartment between AC and NYC, a quarter mile off the ocean. It was during this time in New Jersey that I became close to my Grandma's cousin John and his beautiful Greek family, who had never come west to North Dakota. What a treat to find relatives in my new home! One September morning, as I stood in the hall of WPUR/ Atlantic City, I heard a scream from the traffic department. I rushed into the office to see a plane fly into the South Tower of the World Trade Center. The other tower was already burning. We watched with the rest of the nation as people fell to their fate. But my job was not in the traffic office.

"What's happening?" I shouted to the afternoon guy as he ran past down the hall.

'Hell's breaking loose,".he yelled back.

'Joe wants you in the studio. Now."

We were country music radio personalities. We learned how to be disaster communicators that day. We spent thirteen hours on the air, swallowing our emotions to remain calm, answering the phone and updating the list of closures. I announced when the towers fell. I asked our newsfeed guy if that was a real report, and then I repeated it, louder for our listenership. That night, we piped in the news from the president's rose garden news conferences. Praise God for the peace He granted me. It isn't always clear why we are where we are. I think the best policy is to be thankful when we find ourselves in situations where there is possibility to be helpful.

There is always possibility.

For weeks, I spent nights on the couch in front of my television set with the news on, waiting for another person to be pulled from the wreckage of the World Trade Center. The plastic-smelling cloud of ash from the buildings' collapse had blown downshore, into town, and out again.

Isaiah 40:31 "Yet those who wait for the Lord will gain new strength; they will mount up with wings like eagles, they will run and not get tired, they will walk and not become weary."

I love that verse from Isaiah. Someday, *I* will run and not get tired. *I* will walk and not become weary! It will be sooner than later. A preacher in San Antonio said, "Difficult times do not come to stay. They come to pass."

10/27/01
I called Tyler's mother tonight. Tyler was in the

room across the hall from me in the hospital. He was ten, and had a malignant brain tumor, which could not be removed, even with two surgeries. His recovery took so much longer than mine.

"Sometimes I feel guilty," I told my mom. I felt guilty that other families in the hospital's waiting room would be hoping for a miracle, and wouldn't get one, but I was recovering by leaps and bounds.

"Don't you ever feel guilty for God's miracles!" she said.

I kept in touch with Kathy, Tyler's mother, every few months to see how it was going. Tyler was walking, Tyler was going to half-days of school, and Tyler would be thirteen this fall.

Tyler died Monday. He slipped quietly away in his sleep, at home. He had deteriorated again so quickly, after a brief rise in his condition. His skullosaurus just would not be conquered.

I lay on my living room floor and sobbed until my neighbor Basia knocked on the door, to invite me to dinner to hear about her new business.

I believed in order to get better I needed to exercise my mind as well as my body. How do you maintain a happy disposition? Practice thinking happy thoughts as much as possible.

"Look! The sun is shining!"

"Doesn't that rain smell good?"

I sing in the car a lot.

There is no convenient coffee shop between my apartment and the radio station. I have taken up the habit of making my own coffee in the morning. It takes a little more time, but I also feel more centered, and I saved quite a bit of money that way.

I smile and say hello to every person I see, even though that's not the norm. But if you are friendly at the post office or grocery store, people will remember you, and you will always get good service.

For my birthday that year, my parents drove to New Jersey and hauled me back to San Antonio. I went to work selling and designing ads for the Military Newspapers. It was kind of fun, even though it didn't pay much. Soon, through a friend, I accepted a position at The SCOOTER Store. It would be one of my biggest blessings.

CHAPTER ELEVEN

In the first five years after the surgery, I had just three seizures, overnight and in my sleep. I knew about them, because I would wake up sore with a tremendous headache, sometimes with a severely bitten tongue.

Then I got married. Within two years, I'd had lots of grand mal seizures, during the day, in front of people. That really bothered me, because I didn't ever want anyone to see that. The petit mal seizures make up another hundred. I would color-code them on the calendar, whether they were serious Simple-Complex seizure, or a Complex Partial Onset seizure, just an Absence, or Grand Mal, Tonic-Clonic. They would happen at work.

One took hold of me for forty-five minutes while shopping on a Sunday after church. That one really hurt. I hit my head hard that time. Phyllis, the checkout lady, followed me around the store whenever I went into the store after that, just to make sure I got out again, conscious and intact. Her husband had seizures, and she is hyper vigilant, and a darling lady.

Summer of 2006
The scar tissue from that big tumor had taken seven years to interfere with the rest of my brain. Dr. Luther says scar tissue in the brain is like naughty children on the playground. It tries to get the other children (healthy tissue) to be naughty, too.

I had many seizures and I visited several neurologists in the greater San Antonio area. It could have been stress; it could have been scar tissue. Finally, after the wearing down of two years and several different medications, I expressed to my doctor that I needed this crazy lifestyle to end. I wasn't supposed to drive for six months after a seizure, per Texas law. My seizures were happening twice a week, and once, three times in a day, and I was apprehensive every moment. I wasn't driving then. The seizure disorder had very nearly taken over my life, and the lives of everyone around me. Seizure days left me worn out, dizzy, and confused. Seizure days were rough, and they were the norm. Thank God for my excellent coworkers and friends. They picked me up for work and drove me home. They included me in all of our work and social gatherings, and did not leave me alone. Blessed doesn't begin to cover how I feel about them.

Sooner or later, my medical care team decided to catch one on video. Twenty-seven wires were glued to my head, waiting for convulsions. Ironically, I had a big, painful grand mal at home the morning before checking in, so they didn't get to measure that one.

There was no Internet access, and I was tethered to a video cart which records me, while they do an EEG, waiting. They were hoping to study my brainwaves and find out where in my brain these seizures were coming from. Dr. Bogaev popped in, to see how it was going, to cheer my bored, lonely self up, and to tell me he wants to strive for perfection with me, and get me seizure- and medication-free for the rest of my life. If we could get there, I could drive again. I could run to the store alone. Without the seizures, I wouldn't feel housebound. At this point, I am completely stationary. I cannot go anywhere alone. I am afraid every moment of every day that I'm going to drop and lose consciousness. The hospital did catch a seizure on video. It takes strobe lights, sleep-deprivation, and medication deprivation to do so. But then they watch it and measure it. I was able to watch the beginning of said seizure in Dr. Luther's office. Seeing myself go into convulsions, I had a seizure at his desk.

I was getting organized, to clear my head. I had cleared up my files at work, to make my desk "easy to read" for my coworkers. I cleaned my house, in case the house would be sold, or to prepare for any company. I threw out all old diaries, love poems, letters and musings of old boyfriends. By the morning of August 28, 2006, my parents had driven down to Texas from North Dakota. We arrived at the hospital before 5:00 a.m., and I was not allowed to have coffee that morning. Part of me wanted to exclaim that part (NO COFFEE!), but the rest of me never, ever questions what Dr. Bogaev says. If a man cuts open your head and carefully closes it back up, I think you can put coffee off until, like noon. I was pretty sleepy, and that probably got me through any pre-operative jitters. They did not shave my entire head this time. They shaved one strip down the middle of my head, and two little spots for the sensors, before doing the pre-op MRI.

As we were walking down a hallway toward the registration desk, a loud, "Good morning!" boomed from behind, and we turned around. Army Chaplain Jim Benson, in full battle dress uniform, was following. He had gotten up early to be there. At this point, I was not afraid for me. I know what's out there. I was praying, and tears quietly rolling down the sides of my face as they rolled me into the OR, because now someone is counting on me. It's not just me anymore. I was praying God would be with my family, and I was so very glad Chaplain Jim had come.

Two and a half hours later, my parents were at the foot of my ICU bed, shaking me awake.

"Okay, okay, I'm ready for brain surgery," I mumbled.

"You're done," Dad informed me. "It's over!"

"Done?" I asked. "Well, I told you it'd be easy."

I awoke from my operation feeling like I could conquer the world, and I wanted to. I was ready to start businesses, travel, run marathons, buy land, and fulfill every dream I ever had. There had been no stained glass door this time. I really didn't think I would make it through another brain operation. I had taken the time to look into my insurance beneficiaries and 401K, etc., but who survives two brain surgeries? Especially after the two convulsive years I had just had? I thought I was out of here, that I would be airlifted to Heaven just as soon as the anesthetist got to me. I didn't think I would need to worry anymore about pollution, weight gain, IRA accounts, or the coffee stains on my teeth. Now that I'm apparently indestructible, I need to start making plans!

Jeremiah 29:11
For I know the plans I have for you," declares the LORD, "plans to prosper you and not to harm you, plans to give you hope and a future."

This surgery was completely unlike the last one. They went through the same incision, but I was out of the hospital in just five days. That was a welcome improvement from the two-month stay seven years ago! All of my parts moved, and I was walking around the nurses' station with a walker and a physical therapist within two days. I was feeling pretty motivated by that. Going into this experience, I knew that I didn't want my family to have to go through a lot. I can do whatever I have to, when I have to do it. But I knew that as soon as my eyes opened, I would do my best to dive back into living and get back to work.

Thank God this one came out so well. I feel better than I have in nearly ten years. My friends who have known me all my life and my mother say that they feel like they have the old me back. We decided that if one brain surgery can alter the personality and make a person quieter, perhaps more shy, with downcast eyes, a second operation can change them right back. Makes perfect sense to me!

Genesis 15:15
You, however, will go to your father's in peace and be buried at a good old age.

2/7/2008

I saw Dr. Bogaev this week. I haven't had a seizure in a year and a half. Due to my high energy level and my clarity of mind, he said he wouldn't torture me with another MRI until 2010, if I promise to stop in once in a while. It looks like I have finally reached that day. My "hero surgeon" is asking me to come around, just to keep in touch. I am perfect again. I am tremendously blessed. It was something that happened long, long ago, and not so far away.

There is so much to do now that I'm not having seizures anymore. Other people need help.

My friend Stephanie and I started a financial education nonprofit, to help people get themselves out of debt. It has become more of a conversation starter, or something to talk about at dinner. People ask me how to get themselves out of the painful debt cycle, so I explain it, and it only takes a minute.

"How do I get out of debt?" a coworker, or a friend will

ask me, out of nowhere. "Stop spending so much money," I tell them.

"Thanks," and I get an eye roll.

"No, really. Put your credit cards away. Put yourself on an allowance. Consolidate your car trips. Cook at home. Take your lunch to work. Wash your clothes instead of dry-cleaning them.

It's pretty simple, once you put it on paper and stick to it. And to think, ten years ago, I was in so much trouble, because my brain was swirling.

8/20/2010

My momma used to tell me, "If you're hungry, you can eat. If you're tired, you can sleep. If you are homesick, there is nothing you can do about it."

I want to go home. I love Texas, but I cannot face another Christmas afternoon, taking down my few decorations early, with a Christmas movie marathon on some cable channel while I call home every five minutes asking, "What are you guys doing now? How about now? Did you make the caramels? Did you make the Mexican wedding cakes? How did Grandma look this morning? Is everybody okay?"

I need to be in North Dakota. I need to be doing my part

for my state, my great-great grandfather's legacy, and whatever may come. One of my best friends died of her long cancer battle a few weeks ago, and in the last days, I sat at her bedside, holding her hand and staring into her eyes, assuring her that Heaven is there. It will only be frightening for a moment, before she steps onto the crunchy grass. Liz embodied loveliness. She made every room she was in nicer for everyone around her. Never was a teacup empty, a napkin crumpled, or a face without a smile, if Liz was in attendance.

One day one of my pseudo-grandmothers from church, Martha, took me to a precious tearoom in the Texas Hill Country outside of San Antonio. Its wallpaper charmed me, its porcelain dolls on the high shelves, and its touches of elegance and sheer sweetness. Its owner was a lady named Liz, who had been diagnosed with cancer only a month before. As we were leaving, she stopped me at the door.

'Excuse me," Liz said. "I have to tell you, there is something about your aura. Your eyes just sparkle. You are amazing. I just know we're going to be friends." And we were.

Liz and I drank gallons and gallons of iced tea and coffee, and talked about Heaven and husbands. She'd had four. When I lost my radio gig to a computer, it was Liz who picked me up from the station at midnight, and

Liz who kept my heavy trophy container for the year I lived in New Jersey. When I got married and bought a house in New Braunfels, Liz was very relieved, because she believed that meant I was finally going to settle down and stay. She was sure then, that we were going to be friends forever. And we were.

Ten years later, I sat at her bedside as her organs failed, reminding her what a beautiful life she had, pondering what Heaven would be like, and what to tell Baby Hannah, after she passed.

"Liz, you brought up a good family. They will take care of each other. Now that Melly married into the Air Force, she will have other military wives to lean on, to help her with the baby. I am probably going to go be near my family soon."

BACK HOME TO FARGO

I wouldn't say I was "settled" into my new apartment. My friends Dennis, Carrie, Greg and I got the moving truck emptied and everything stuffed into the place. Carrie and Greg went to a matinee, and Dennis and I went to drop off the moving truck at the rental place before hitting Perkins, a local diner, to have breakfast for dinner. He's got to have potato pancakes.
My parents dropped by later on their way through town and Dad and Dennis assembled my new couch. I had

seating once again in my living room! After my divorce in Texas, I had systematically erased every bit of furniture from my home. I even sold the dishes on a garage sale, and donated the proceeds to my Relay For Life team.

When everybody left, I hunkered down and slept with the lights on. This feeling was familiar. I was surrounded by boxes in an apartment. I could have been anywhere. It might well have been Atlantic City. Sometimes I wake in the morning and forget which city I'm living in.

When I awoke, I could feel and see the difference in the daylight. It wasn't normal daylight, coming in the window of my new bedroom. I sat up in my bed and turned around. The window was completely glazed over by Jack Frost's handiwork.

"No, no, no, NO!" I actually cried out loud. I hurried to the patio door in the kitchen, and slid it open to find big, gorgeous flakes fluttering from Heaven. To my shock and amazement, there was at least one foot of fluffy snow. If I was shocked and amazed, Lucky was completely flabbergasted. One of the most precious sights I have ever seen, is my Siberian Husky's first snow interaction. She was born in Texas, and never knew this kind of precipitation was possible.

The Texan in me was sure this was a dream, and if I just went back to sleep, it would be melted away by noon. I didn't have cable, internet, or groceries. And I was COLD. There were boxes everywhere, but I did have an assembled sofa. I could not even locate my coffeemaker, and the headache was beginning to creep in and become frightening to me. I had to raise caffeine, and FAST. I called Carrie, good, reliable Carrie from college, who had already scoped out my needs from my apartment complex. Carrie has a map of Fargo in her brain.

"Exit your complex," Carrie said. "Go through that stop sign. One block and the grocery store's on your right."

I have amazing friends. They will take care of me.

Pushing a grocery cart across a parking lot in a foot of snow, while it's still coming down in gargantuan flakes is no small feat. I happened to select the cart with the wonky wheel. You know the one. It's at your grocery store, too, and you fight with it all the way through to the checkout. Now try pushing that through a snow drift.

I should have tied Lucky to it and MUSHED right on through! I have no doubt these are acquired skills, or perhaps cell memory can assist me with this, but this is why Dakotans live here-- because no one else can.

There are four distinct seasons. Three are beautiful, and one is very distinct. It just so happens that in November, when I was visiting Fargo, that longer-than-normal autumn was a ruse. This, this is winter. And this winter MEANS IT.

CHAPTER TWELVE

WHAT I LEARNED FROM THE BRAIN TUMOR

Take care of yourself! I have great blood pressure and blood sugar and perfect vision. I eat a lot of vegetables. Doc has me on some fancy-smancy diet now, where I don't eat bread anymore. Eventually, you don't miss it. I still have a hitch in my giddyup (my friend Dana's compassionate way of saying "limp"), but I am free to live and love my community. Isn't that what we all want for our lives and each other?

My friends who know me well don't notice the gait disturbance, and it seems to be the first thing new people notice about me. That doesn't bother me a lot, because I am acquainted with enough loving people, that the insulting remarks are a drop in the bucket. I don't have an overabundance of time to think about my left leg. There is still so much to do

For example, a meningioma in your Hypothalamus hooks you up with all kinds of animated emotions, if you weren't a bit of a drama queen prior to this (I was The Communications, Speech and Theatre Association of North Dakota Best Actress of 1994, thank you very much). Be careful, though. Strong emotions can be a seizure trigger.

Sometimes the people seem to be a little put off by someone who is never in a bad mood, and has a gait disturbance. Maybe it's the anti-seizure maintenance med, which is also used as a mild antidepressant. NEWSFLASH: I've always been like this. I've been cheerful since kindergarten. I have solid references.

Perhaps, and this is just a shot in the dark, maybe I'm just on a real reality trip, and I'm real thankful to be walking, talking, and independently feeding myself. I can work, live, drive, frequent my favorite coffee shop, talk on the phone, take myself to the bathroom, and go to the refrigerator without having to wait for someone to push my wheelchair away from The Feeding Group. Maybe all this constant Pathological Pleasantry is a tangible gift from the Lord, and I am not wasting a drop of it.

I was lost. Now I'm found. Praise God my chains are gone.

I thought the further away from that tumor I got, the better I would get. I have days during which I am perfect. Most days I am amazing. Some days I have to drag myself out of bed and through the door and I do not know why. Some days things actually hurt, from the top of my head to the tips of my toes, and I can't figure that one out. These are typically days when the temperature gauge reads many tens of degrees below zero.

I suppose I should migrate back to the South more often. My last fifteen years has taught me that you really do need to listen to your breathing. Be very grateful for every breath, and every heartbeat. Understand what a miracle it is that you can walk across a room, or run a marathon. The human body can do so much, yet sometimes it takes so little to damage is forever. Be very kind to everyone, because we are all making our journey at our own speed. Be ready to get here when you get there, not a moment later and not a moment too soon.

After a frustrating day, I am driving along. It's one of those roads. There's one in every town. It's a little bit longer with fewer traffic lights, and it is a little newer than some of the other streets, so it feels like a racetrack.

As my wheels ka-chunk, ka-chunk over the lines in the road, I ka-chunk, ka-chunk talk to God.

"What can I do, Lord? Change me so I have a better disposition or more compassion with this situation. I don't feel very patient right now."

I talk out loud to God in my car. He's used to it, and it works for us. He doesn't mind my singing.

"Show me what to do. Where do I need to go? How can I help? What am I supposed to be doing?"

The answer came back so crystal clearly. It rang out like a bell just as I crossed a bridge over a beautiful golf course and the blue sky calmly dwelt above manicured greens begging for play.

"You don't have to do anything. Just BE."

My breath caught in my throat as I realized I had really just heard what I thought I had just heard. When I started breathing again, tears fell off my jawline as quickly as they poured from my eyes. God wasn't telling me to stop doing all of the things I enjoy. I don't have to stay home or forget about my schedule of volunteerism. He was telling me that I could stop worrying about whether any of it was making a difference. Each of us does our part, we contribute our gifts, and then thanks to Gestalt psychology, the whole is greater than the sum of its parts.

I could stop fretting over people liking me or not liking me. Other peoples' bad days are not my fault. I simply could be His child. He created me with this journey and these gifts. He must have something in mind for it.

7/2015

UFFDAH, as the Norwegians say in Minnesota. Parts of me think I'm getting older. My heart does not agree. It could be arthritis settling into my back. Last fall, I was an administrative assistant at an office, which handles a public form of insurance. My supervisor realized that, as a multi-tasker, I needed more to keep busy, so he had me inventory the entire department and prepare for the office move to a new location.

This did not win me friends. When the time came to pack the files into fifty-two paper boxes, no one could take time away from their instant messaging and online shopping, and I packed all of it.

Keeping in mind that my left side is weak and my balance is poor, I packed, sealed, labeled, stacked, hauled down a hallway, and restacked fifty years' worth of public insurance history, legislative bills, laws, meeting notes and old printed out emails.

Upon reaching the new location, I asked for help to refile all of this. I had reached my physical limit, I told my manager. I could not reach. I could not lift one more 50-pound box of paper. He told me to do what I could do, and left for an all-day meeting.

I eventually sat down when a coworker brought me her project. I said I would try to help her with it in the morning.

"No," she said. "You will do it now."

I was surprised at first by her tone, so I laughed. ThenI was awed. She was serious. I tried to be really honest with myself. Maybe I was being a little weak. I unpacked it and refiled all of it. Until something snapped/tore/strained and my body informed me I would do no more of this.

I woke up the next morning with a burning spine, and the burning sensation extended across the top of my back, to my shoulders and down my arms. My hands were both numb.

The director of the department was back in the office from his meeting. He had me fill out an incident report and called the risk manager, who sent me to the doctor immediately. They later informed me my position was eliminated.

That afternoon the doctor said my neck and lumbar were sprained. MRI scans would show a torn right rotator cuff. Given the memories of my times past in the hospital relearning all that I had, I was afraid.My position eliminated. In addition to my weak left side, this was unhandy. My left hand was more useless than usual, and now my right hand shook all the time. I couldn't hold anything. And that was the last time I would ever succumb to bullying.

In the months to come, I would do intense, and sometimes painful, physical therapies until I would cry, traction most days, and massage on others. I would have difficulty getting dressed and brushing my hair. I would be unable to carry my purse or write my own name. If I wanted to cook or bake something, I would invite the neighbors over to handle the pans for me, because I couldn't lift them.

For a long time, I could only drink the smallest cup of coffee at a time. A larger cup triggers some very painful and uncomfortable muscles in my upper right arm and upper back, and I could not get a sip of coffee without a drastic tremor. On one occasion, I was out for lunch with my parents, and they were observing my crazy system of trying to navigate anything to my mouth. My right arm was shaking so badly with pain, that I had to steady it with my left hand, which usually shakes uncontrollably.

I'm using my right hand, because I'm right handed, and I help with my hemiplegic left hand, for strength. My arms begin to burn quickly. I can't talk on the phone longer than about two minutes.

It's not a cut-and-dried, 90-degree life. But we find a workaround when we have to. .

Fall 2015
Above and beyond all of the discomfort, and the kind of weird-sounding intricacies of what it's like to have parts of your body you have to keep checking on to make sure they haven't fallen off of the planet somewhere, this is pretty good.
I became a Number One Bestselling Author on Amazon, for co-authoring The Energy of Happiness. A month later, I was blessed to work with that group of co-authors again and we became Two-Time Number One Bestselling Authors on Amazon, with the release of The Energy of Receiving.

I have, by being home in North Dakota, been able to spend cherished time with my family. I am joyful that I was near when Mom went through cancer treatment, and I am more than exuberant that she is doing very well.

Thanks to Grandma's love of storytelling, and my love of sharing in that with her, I have three historical fictions on the shelves. Something About Sophia honors my pioneering great-great grandmother, and Nowhere, Everywhere explores the adventurous girl inside all of us. Love And War: Timeless shares the passing down of compassion from one's Greatest Generational grandparents. I believe we all have lessons we can glean from any interaction with our elders.

CHAPTER THIRTEEN

I was sixteen the first time lightning got too close to my body. My friend Jill and I were walking down a street in our small town, late at night, in the summer, and we could smell the rain.

We were giggling about shopping. Weighing the better investment, jeans or shirts, and very, very suddenly, the flash hit the street in front of us. The memory of it takes my breath away. I flinched. Jill did not. She couldn't see for a few minutes, but she grabbed my arm and yelled. "We have to hide under the tree!" I pulled her back, because I didn't know if any of the nearby trees would topple over, due to what had just occurred. Jill's house was a block away. We had to get there.

All of this seemed to take a very long time, but it was seconds. The loudest crack of thunder I'd ever heard popped over the tops of our heads. Across town, Suzy was writing a check at the gas station, and scratched her pen across the counter. That crack from her pen was there for years.

The rainshower erupted as Jill and I scampered into her house. She wasn't dazed anymore from the lightning, so we watched a movie.

It wasn't until the next day that we noticed the face on my watch was shattered.

At twenty-one, I had probably the coolest job among all of my college friends. I was a radio deejay. Granted, I had to work some Saturdays, but I still got free concert tickets. The station at which I worked had several large dishes in the parking lot.

The time was coming up on 3:00. I gave the weather report. Thirty percent chance of storms in the area. Without any more warning than that, and a quick, ear-to-ear ZAP(!) through my headphones, the Spice Girls were gone from my airspace. I was a little dazed, as you are if you hit your head on something and it stings for just a minute.

After about two minutes, we were brought back on air. Two of the gentlemen who worked on the AM station walked in just as the station came live on the air again, rushed into my control room, and excitedly informed me there was a dead, black, charred squirrel outside in the parking lot, and I would have to take a look when my shift was over. Imagine that.

Two years later, almost immediately following my brain tumor removal, I began to have what I described as, "Lightning Pains." I told scant few people about these sensations at the time, because I didn't want them to think I was losing my mind. I also didn't want them to get tired of hearing me complain all of the time. People can only take so much.

A couple of years ago, I asked my dad what these lightning pains might be.

"Maybe you'll just have to make friends with it," he'd offered.

Fair enough. If nothing can be done, and you've got to cope, the best thing to do, is paint on your smile and hope. These small bolts of electricity rumbled across my right eyebrow and cheekbone pretty continuously.

132

I've "made friends" with the sensation of Trigeminal Neuralgia, as I just accepted it would never change. Moments would pass with tingly waves across my right eyebrow and cheekbone. Perhaps it was a breeze. Sometimes I thought a fly landed on my face. Always, I would brush it away. These moments became more common and the tingles became more like lightning bolts. They were very fast, almost pin prickly, and by the time my hand reached up to brush the pain away, the storm had passed. Such a storm leaves in its wake a rumbling, sometimes swollen path, in this case, my right eye.

So many days, Mom would sit across the bistro table from me wherever we happened to be having coffee and observe, "Your eye is red. Did you sleep last night?"

Several of those days, my manager at work would ask if I was crying, but retract her inquiry, because only one eye was red. It's just so weird. It doesn't even look like allergies. Fast forward.

Yes, please fast forward. Through nineteen years and another brain surgery and dozens of seizures and laser eye correction, so I don't have to put contact lenses in that eye anymore.

Even when you make friends with your neuralgia, or

lightning pains, they arrive unannounced. Even when you tell your crazy nerve pain, "Look, hey, I get it. You're here, you're frantic, and you're going to rear your ugly head all over my head. Can you chill a little?"

I made friends with the lightning pains, but our relationship is stormy. Sometimes it knocks me dizzy. Sometimes it knocks me deaf. Once in a while, it knocks me daft. I forget what I'm saying, to whom I'm speaking, and what I'm doing. I don't want to explain to everyone, every time, that I just had a flash of lightning across my face. These days, the Lightning zaps have moved into my ears and behind my right eye. It's surprising every time it happens, and keeps every day interesting. I try to maintain composure.

The neurologist says he cannot do anything about this. I'm already taking the maximum dosage of what they would prescribe for neuralgia, for my seizure risk, so I've just got to use my super-rock steady coping skills. This is where deep breathing, light yoga, and faith come in.

CHAPTER FOURTEEN

My doctor said the words, "I can't do anything else for you. I can send you to a higher clinic somewhere else, like Mayo, or maybe Cleveland." For one breath I processed his words. People get sent to Mayo Clinic when they're really sick or have cancer. I have never considered my journey as fearful or life-threatening, because my life will continue in Heaven. My verbal response?

"Send me back to Texas."

Dr. recommended a few various options. I could try The Ketogenic Diet. I could try Botox (It's supposed to help some people), or we could switch up my meds. Switching up my meds almost always leads to seizures for me, so he said we should get prepared for disability. It takes a lot of work to prove one is disabled. My doctor said they would never believe I was disabled because I present so well. I told him I don't believe in wearing illness. He sent me for a neuropsych evaluation. A what? Am I crazy?

No. This is just an evaluation to see what damage the scar tissue is doing to me outwardly. It is a necessary piece of the puzzle for disability approval. Okay, got it. The results were pretty clear. Dr. Swenson informed me and my parents that had the meningioma been on the other side of my brain, I would not be able to remember my name, let alone anything else. He also said it was time for me to go on disability. Nineteen years in the workforce after the event was long enough. After seizures, I have days' worth of verbal setbacks. Stress is not good for me. Being medically retired would be good for my health.

September 2017
I had another seizure at work. It was a long one, fifteen minutes, and it scared my coworkers. A wobbly, sore week follows. Why it happened, no one knows. I'm thankful for good family nearby. I couldn't remember much or text on my phone for about three days. I'm blessed my parents could pick me up from the emergency room. One of the paramedics is from my hometown.

What is super important to me (super important is like regular important, but with a cape, y'all), is that I don't get sidelined from the 5K I've been working toward.

Here I am, already two days out of seizure, and my headache is still so bad I can hear the bruises holler to each other from my temples, past the blown veins in my eyes, from my last Emergency Room visit a few months ago.

I'm having a little trouble reading, a lot of trouble walking, and no trouble praying. Thank God for my good, good family. I have best friends in my cousins and brothers, who are well trained in how to handle seizures. And my parents? Pretty incredible.

Two weeks after a fifteen-minute grand mal, I turned the corner and saw it: The Finish Line at The Bismarck Marathon 5K. I had been walking for nearly three miles, and we had almost half a mile to go. My parents' dear friend from their high school days, Shelly, registered and walked with me. She's a teacher, and walks far further than 5 kilometers daily. She wasn't about to have me get lost or hurt on the three-mile route somewhere, winding through the park.

I had twisted my left ankle somewhere around Mile Two. I hollered back and told those sunshiny faces I was so happy they were there.

Closer to our destination, the race announcer standing beneath his pop-up tent. He asked me my name.

"Josie Blaine, for the American Brain Tumor Association!" I showed him my blue Team Breakthrough shirt. He repeated the words over the loudspeakers. My fundraising efforts and the beautiful hearts around me had brought in $500 in the weeks prior to the race! I heard my name over the loudspeaker. Then I looked forward, asking, "Where's my mom?" over and over, scanning the crowd along the orange snow fence. Someone was yelling for me.

"You have to cross the finish line!" Kory, from my

church, waiting for her marathoner husband, Dave, was beckoning me that I had about thirty feet to go. "Come on! You have to cross the finish line!"

I almost collapsed laughing. But I limped across the finish line at The Bismarck Marathon 5K.

CHAPTER FIFTEEN

The seizures are back. They're so ugly.

Remember that neurologist from May of 2001? Well, Dr. Bogaev sent me back to him. The appointment took five months to schedule, because their program is growing and they're one of the top neurology/seizure/TBI research centers in Texas. Good. Fix me. During that five month wait, I had tonic-clonic seizures and simple-partial seizures and tried to sleep enough, but none of us could figure it out. I flew down and stayed with my brother and sister-in-love.

Not long after arrival, I had a half hour of seizures in Trav's living room, for several minutes of which I was conscious but not breathing. That was new. I could hear the gurgling in my throat. I could feel my body shaking, ever so slightly. My brother has informed me that over the years my seizures have changed, and I don't really have big convulsions like I used to. My jaw was locked and I was staring at the ceiling fan. I heard Travis talking to me, telling me it was time to call EMS.

I realized I hadn't been breathing for a while, and prayed to lose consciousness. I figured, while in that state, he could handle it. Within what seemed like a blink, it was something like 5:30 in the morning, and there was my brother, sitting at my side in the Emergency Room. As soon as I was conscious enough for the doctor to talk to me and receive feedback, they let us go home.

I was bummed that this year I was missing my Brain Tumor 5K, so I did an online fundraiser for the American Brain Tumor Association. There has got to be some more research done. They have to figure out what causes these menaces, which hide within the skull, changing a personality and a life, eventually breaking hearts. Speaking of research, I was about to check into the research hospital for this study on my head. Hopefully it helps someone.

San Antonio was flooding the morning we were supposed to go in to the hospital. My brother's car was flooded up to the seats. Good thing he has a truck. We had to fjord down the street to where his truck was parked.

When I got to the hospital, they wired my head with those 27 wires again and took me off my medication. I went to sleep at ten.

They woke me up at 2:00 a.m.

They made me ride a bike for two hours nonstop.

Then, at 7:30a.m., every morning, the strobe light people came in. They flashed me in the face with different frequencies of a strobe light for four hours. Eventually, the seizures came.

Big, ugly, painful, muscle-tightening, tongue-biting 30-minute seizures in two days, just like they wanted. Three seizures in three weeks slows me down physically and sometimes verbally for a few weeks, but with a few sessions of physical therapy I'll be back at it. They got them recorded on video. I don't know what it means yet. I get the results of all that in four months. More medication for now. Hopefully safety. Seems like we're going to try anything.

I remember leading the Halloween River Parade my first year in San Antonio. I remember dancing the night away as I hostessed dance parties on the Riverwalk on the radio. I remember the first day I was lifted to my feet in the rehabilitation hospital, and I had a sense of standing again. I remember the Sunday I first stood up from my wheelchair at Main Post Gift Chapel when Renee, our worship director, asked us to turn our hymnals to, "Stand Up, Stand Up, for Jesus."

I remember walking four steps with a walker in the therapy gymnasium of Warm Springs Rehabilitation Hospital in San Antonio, TX, then eight. Then sixteen. I remember the day I walked three miles to raise five hundred dollars for brain tumor research, and almost forgot to cross the Finish Line.

Every single time, my momma cried. Let's keep going, friends. Don't forget your finish line.

Make every day a blessed one for yourself and your family. Travel. Have a coffee. Eat good food. Make plans and get excited, because it's good for your heart.

Hug somebody. Send out love. Don't forget your finish line, and know someone is waiting for you there.

Made in the USA
Monee, IL
24 April 2024

57462671R00079